BREAKING THE CHAINS OF OBESITY

107 TOOLS

Jennifer Zerling, MS, CPT

ISBN: 1466469900
ISBN-13: 9781466469907

NOTICE

This book was written in nontechnical language for the general reader. It is intended to be a reference only and is not intended to be a medical manual. The information given here is designed to guide you through your weight-loss journey. It is not intended to be a substitute for any treatment or advice that has been prescribed by your doctor. If you suspect that you have a medical problem, we advise that you talk to your doctor today before embarking on any of the aspects of the plan in this book.

This book is not written to supplement or replace any other sound practices that have been advised by your primary caregiver. All parts of this book may have inherent risks, including the tips that involve physical activity or nutritional guidance. The writer, editor, and publisher advise readers to take full responsibility for their own safety and know their own limits, and remove themselves from any and all liability. As with any information that is intended for weight loss, you should get your primary care physician's approval before beginning.

Mention of specific companies, organizations, or authorities in this book does not imply endorsement by the author or

CONTENTS

ACKNOWLEDGMENTS

Thank you for purchasing my book. I love that you want to better yourself, and I'm flattered that you chose to read my words.

Thank you, G&S Sporting Goods (www.GSboxing.com), for your sponsorship of this book. Thank you, Dad, for making me the athlete I am today. My two siblings and I are grateful for the competitive edge you've instilled in us.

Thank you, Mom, for inspiring me every day to work hard at everything I do. You're an amazing friend, excellent listener, and the most fabulous mother a girl can ever dream of. Thank you for discovering the perfect book title and for your help with editing.

Grandma Sylvie, thank you so much for always taking my phone calls at two in the morning, New York time. Our conversations always inspire me. I am forever grateful to you. I can't wait to read your book, Grandma! Your life experience is such an amazing lesson plan for us all.

Catarina, thank you for being an amazing friend to me. Your sisterhood has taught me charisma, sexiness, and confidence. Thank you for being a terrific therapist for those who need someone great to care about them. You've mastered this.

Randy, thank you for being an amazing brother and for being a smart and talented young man. Your personal drive in your career is always inspiring to me. It's an honor to say that you are my bro.

Thank you, Alan, for all the therapy for my shoulders and back after sitting endlessly to write this book. You will be the best chiropractor and husband in the world. Your ongoing support is invaluable to me. I love you so much. Rana and Howie Fecher, thank you for giving me the most amazing son to travel in my journey of life with!

Thank you, Dino Sergi (www.dinosergi.com), for the beautiful book cover photography; Neda Keshavarz, for being my unofficial personal assistant; and Jason Savitt from www.verticalinterval.com for producing my JZ fitness reel.

Thank you, Shirin Farahani (www.shirinsalon.com), for doing my hair and makeup for every photo shoot even if it meant waking up at six a.m. on a Saturday morning.

Thank you, Shane Bell (www.bellmakeup.com), for the awesome internal photos (except for tool #85 shot by my girl Xochitl Rodrigue from www.thexgallery.com); Thank you, Khan, at www.99designs.com for my JZ Fitness logo and Lauren Moshi (www.laurenmoshi.com) for providing me with your artistic expertise. You rock!

Meg Tomczak Mongell, thank you for being an amazing friend and for our annual goal-review sessions. Thank you, Nancy Sharpe, for watching Bebe when I'm on the road.

Thank you, Dr. Roman Lal, for your belief in my expertise and for supporting my writing of this book. It's an honor to work with you. Thank you, Brandi Reed, for your support while writing this book; and Dr. Yvonne Maywether, for teaching me new things about medicine when we talk.

Dr. Patricia Sherblom, you are great for all the years of advising me and believing in my expertise even beyond my graduation from my masters program.

Thank you, Garry Grant and Brad Lipschultz at SEO Inc. (http://www.seoinc.com), for building my blog site, www.JZfitness.com. Without SEO, I wouldn't have such an amazing site.

Thank you, Bud Knapp, for all our pep talks and for caring about my success so much!

Gosh, I hope I didn't forget anyone. I feel like I'm on stage at the Academy Awards. I love so many people that I should write another book just thanking everyone who has blessed me in my life. You all know who you are. Thank you!

FOREWORD

Obesity in the United States, the Western world, and also in the Middle East has reached more than epidemic levels. Up to 25 to 35 percent of adults are obese, and an astonishing number of children are too. Hand in hand with the increase in obesity is the development of degenerative diseases such as osteoarthritis, metabolic syndrome with diabetes mellitus type 2, hypertension, and hyperlipidemia with all its consequences such as coronary artery disease, generalized atherosclerosis, and strokes. Moreover, obesity is now considered a risk factor for the development of heart failure, which affects almost seven million people in the United States alone with five hundred thousand newly diagnosed cases per year. Obesity has taken the lead as a risk factor for several diseases ahead of smoking, substance abuse, and other contributing factors.

In contrast to the fate of organ failure, obesity and its fatal consequences can be controlled and reversed, as long as the individual patients understand the severity of the problem and receive adequate guidance to implement lifestyle changes including dieting and exercising. Thousands of programs and books and dietary plans have failed to achieve long-term results with regard to weight loss, maintenance of reduced weight, and prevention of chronic debilitating diseases caused by obesity. The reasons for these failures are incompletely understood, but professionally guided programs that help to endorse self-discipline as positive motivation with visible results for feedback rather than penalty and struggle are sparse. For that reason I strongly endorse Jennifer Zerling's book *Breaking the Chain of Obesity*, and I am personally impressed by her angle of intervention. She is creative in her strategies, thorough with her explanations, excellent with her follow-up, and brilliant in her knowledge base of the diseases that couple with obesity. She has more passion for people in her industry than I have ever seen before. She has trained me personally with regard to my own diet as well as in the gym. She is amazing at what she does. Anyone who follows her lead is in the right hands.

I have read many books on diets but never endorsed any of those because of the lack of long-term success. Jennifer Zerling's book is different since it takes an approach that teaches the reader "how-to" do the things that are needed for weight loss that empowers each of us to choose a tool we all can use each day to succeed in our weight loss journey. Every tool in this book is sharp as long as the readers believe in themselves and in the journey of change. I strongly support Jennifer's weight-loss approach for a slimmer and healthier time ahead of us.

Ernst R. Schwarz, MD, PhD, FACC, FESC, FSCAI
Chief Medical Officer, Heart Institute of Southern California
Professor of Medicine, Cedars Sinai Medical Center
Professor of Medicine, David Geffen School of Medicine, UCLA

PREFACE

I am part of the first generation in my family to break the chains of obesity! Amazing, right? People look me up and down and always respond with, "You come from an overweight family? How are you so lean?" The answer is yes, I come from a family chain of overweight individuals, and I will explain how I'm lean. The nutritional behaviors we learned as children should have perpetuated another generation of obese people, my two siblings and me. If we had continued eating the same way we did as children, this book would have never been written. So how did we break our chains? Here's the story:

Luckily, I had two athletic parents growing up, and my dad always kept my sister, my brother, and me moving. Every Saturday morning at eight a.m., I would awaken to the resounding noise of his lawn mower starting up right outside my window. I was conditioned to fly out of bed, brush my teeth, put on my sweats, and do the yard work—which I hated! Although yard work was good exercise, my father unfortunately rewarded us with a big hearty breakfast at a restaurant called "Good Times" (oh, were those good times!) You walked into this hole-in-the-wall restaurant that probably would have earned a New York "B" rating for cleanliness because it was nasty inside. The smell of dishwasher soap wafted through the air as you were being seated. You could smell the aroma of greasy bacon, butter, and maple syrup topping these gigantic warm pancakes or waffles. That's what got me excited! My dad would always have me order a large stack of four chocolate chip pancakes topped with tons of whipped cream just so he could reach his fork in and have some. For lunch, we would rummage through the aisles of Costco for free samples. Afterward, he made up for this poor eating by taking us to play baseball or tennis. From there we would frequent a fast-food restaurant where we all ordered a fried chicken sandwich or burger with french fries. Thankfully we were always active as children, but we ate the worst food in the world!

My siblings and I were "thicker" throughout our childhood as a result of this. Of course we were. Both parents worked to help provide us with everything we needed as kids. They are great parents. Mom, before she left for work, always left coupons on the kitchen table for either two large pizza pies (buy one get one free—who can pass on that, especially since it's also New York pizza), fried chicken and biscuits, Chinese food, or chicken parmesan heroes with pasta. Yeah, that was indeed what I used to eat.

So how did I fall into a fitness career? Long story short, I was an athlete and cheerleader growing up. Following that, I attended the University at Albany in New York and was quite inactive for my first two years of college due to high academic demands. I decided not to be a part of the cheerleading squad because it didn't appeal to me. My inactivity caused me to gain twenty pounds my first two years. I was pushing a higher BMI, but didn't allow myself to become officially *overweight*.

During my junior year of college, I joined Bally Total Fitness down the street from school since the campus gym was way too far to walk to in negative-ten-degree weather. During my new member orientation, my trainer, Pablo, and I hit it off and were giggling the entire time. The fitness manager, named

4

Chaz, witnessed our interaction and told me that he liked my animated personality. He wanted to hire me since Bally's was in dire need of a female trainer. I told him that I aspired to be a Broadway star, not a trainer. He proposed that while pursuing my acting career in New York City, I could train. At that point, the seed was planted. I begged my mother for the money for my first certification and then got certified and hired at Bally's. It was actually cool to finish college while landing what I thought back then was a mock career as a personal trainer even though Broadway was my childhood dream.

Working at Bally's prompted me to lose the twenty pounds I gained in college. I still ate badly. I remember Pablo asking me, "You're eating ice cream? You're gonna get fat!" I wanted to fit in so I ditched the cone and grabbed a protein shake. I remember thinking to myself, "Ugh, this is so not the same as an ice cream cone."

In that moment, I felt like a prisoner to my own emotions. I was bored with the shake. That cone was my reward for working a job while juggling an eighteen-credit semester in college, a radio talk show, a sorority, a peer education group, and my acting career. As a nineteen-year-old girl who aspired to be great at everything I did, I sometimes reverted back to my childhood comfort and dove into the divine taste of an ice cream cone. I always wanted to eat whatever I wanted to because that's how I was raised. Food comforted me. Being twenty pounds heavier did not.

I left Bally's after college to perform professionally. I landed an acting job in Vermont and gained my twenty pounds back. After the show, I moved to New York City and worked for New York Sports Clubs (NYSC), where I lost the weight again. As you know, New York has amazing food. The personal trainer health kick went down the tubes from time to time, but as a single girl who didn't want to gain that weight back, I had to behave. I knew back then that partying and eating a sandwich and french fries at four in the morning didn't make me a credible trainer. In order to break the chains of poor eating habits, I needed a much bigger mental and emotional commitment on a *consistent basis*.

Thanks to the Bally's fitness team and my fitness manager, Mike Bailey, from NYSC, I fell in love with the fitness industry. Early in 2001, I was promoted at NYSC to the assistant fitness manager at the Columbus Circle location. This move slowly shifted my time and focus away from acting. The contemplation of a career change cluttered my mind for months. It was a tremendous change for me. I will never forget the day when the answer came forth. I felt terrible for canceling my personal training clients on Wall Street the day before 9/11 for an audition uptown in the theater district. At around 9:10 a.m. on 9/11/01, I called my friend Lee, and he abruptly told me that he couldn't talk because our city was under attack. Every American had a life-shaking experience after that disaster. To this day, I thank my creator for sending me uptown that day since I worked only a block away from Ground Zero. I feel deeply wounded for all the families who lost their loved ones. To this day, I miss my courageous friend John Perry who worked for the New York City Police Department and perished in Tower One during his rescue efforts. This tragic event made me realize that we don't have forever to fulfill our dreams. This is when I decided to take the leap of faith and pursue my dream of living in Los Angeles. The lifestyle that Southern California offered was one in which my heart belonged. Despite the fact that this dream was three thousand miles away from my amazing family, I followed my dream and moved to California back in 2002.

I moved to Los Angeles to pursue a fitness career, not to be an actress. I learned in time that I loved being a fitness expert, and I wholeheartedly committed to this change. I parallel this to any goal that anyone is struggling with. When you want something really badly but there are barriers in your way, it's up to you to power through those barriers by committing to what you really want. That's what I did, and trust me, it wasn't easy-but very rewarding.

I've enjoyed a dynamic journey evolving as a fitness expert over the last ten years through working at high-end health clubs and at medical weight-loss and age-management clinics. I've attended many educational workshops in medicine, fitness, and sports. I have also attained a master's degree in kinesiology. For my thesis, I conducted an innovative study at an elementary school that created a physical education program for an underprivileged school that didn't have one. The program involved a circuit of age-appropriate activities that the children performed at intervals to elevate their heart rates over the course of six weeks. My goal was to reduce body fat levels, which was achieved. The surgeon general continues to warn the public that children must be active and eat right when they're young; otherwise, the likelihood of being an overweight adult is tripled. I am driven to be amongst the others in my industry who are dedicated to fighting against childhood obesity.

The information presented in this book stems from my many years of experience in the fitness and medical fields. The intention of this book is to provide a toolbox of answers to the question of how to get your weight off so that you and your family can be healthy.

If you're ready to open up your mind and dive into the new opportunities ahead of you, then let's get the weight off for real this time!

LET'S BEGIN

This isn't just another weight-loss book. It's an interactive book that's filled with a toolbox of strategies that'll help you along in your weight loss journey.

You must first stop basing your overall success solely on the number you see on the scale. This number is only the result of your behaviors. If the scale doesn't budge, then it's time to check yourself. Never quit on yourself, just check yourself. Open this book up when you need to check yourself and read a tool. Be open-minded so that you can clearly see what needs to shift.

In *Breaking the Chains of Obesity*, there are 107 tools separated into five chapters titled "Uncluttering Your Life," "The Power of Your Mind," "Your Body Is Your Temple," "Motivation to Do It," and "Humanitarianism Can Lift Your Soul." The tools can be mastered one by one and don't have a deadline attached. Read each tool independently from one another and allow the seeds of change to grow in your mind over time. For your convenience, you'll find each tool numbered at the top outside corner of each page. This will provide you with a quick find method for each tool that is referenced throughout the book. Just flip to the tool that I reference if you wish to read about it again. At the end of each tool, you'll find follow up questions listed as exercises that will help you assimilate these tools into your life. I also invite you to visit me on my Web site, www.JZfitness.com, for more JZ love. It's time to bridge the gap between the knowing and the doing.

With that, I give you a toolbox of *how to* successfully lose your weight. Good luck, and have fun acquiring a greater you!

Chapter 1

UNCLUTTERING YOUR LIFE

Uncluttering your life means getting rid of the clutter that distracts you from getting healthier. Clutter has kept you in the dieting cycle for years. If you don't address the root of your problems, then you'll never succeed at long-term weight loss. Clutter keeps you disorganized, which causes you personal chaos. Who can succeed at anything with chaos in their lives? This is why it's time to dump the trash.

TOOL 1. UNCLUTTER YOUR HEAD

A cluttered head does not top a lean body. Get rid of the stress and get organized! I remember my elementary school teachers made us stand alphabetically in a straight line everyday, which was so annoying because I was always last with the letter Z. That was organization. There was no thought involved about where we should stand because we always stood in back of the same person. Easy enough. I mention this because as children, we knew what we needed to do and we did it. This kept us in order. Create order in your day by establishing a daily routine. A daily routine will eventually become automatic for you through consistent efforts. Don't give yourself additional decisions to make when lifestyle decisions should become automatic for you. Being consistent with eating properly, exercising, getting the appropriate amount of sleep, water and managing your stress levels effectively will eventually become routine for you. The way to achieve this is to establish a specific order that you can turn to every day without fail. If going to the gym after work is your daily routine, you must follow through with that plan, the same way I used to be last in line in elementary school.

Start by getting a pen and paper and writing to-do lists. Next, follow through with each item. Start scheduling your workouts and your meal preparations. If you have the funds, then another option is to hire someone to plan this for you and/or help you execute it all. Either way, it is all doable if you really want it. Mounds of mental clutter offer you no time to think about yourself. This is why you can't lose weight. Your to-do-list is the first step to launching you through a successful journey of lifestyle modification. Journaling (tool 28) also helps.

As an adult, you work for a business that has a business plan. Your boss holds you accountable for your work. You're asked to turn in goal sheets. You might have children who count on your leadership every day. You have friends who ask you for favors that you can't say no to. But when it comes to you, you don't commit because the only person you're really disappointing is yourself. Isn't there something wrong with this picture? You manage to always put yourself last, even though last place may never even happen. Your words sound like, "I'll get to the gym later" or "I have no time to eat so I'm just gonna stop and get fast food—just for today." I know what you're all dealing with. It's time to revert to what we learned as children and get organized. Organization helps diminish the overwhelming stressors of the day. Less stress equals more focus. More focus equals being on track with your weight-loss goal.

I remember when I worked at a medical weight-loss facility and signed up a woman for a ten-week program. This woman bought the program because the price was half off at the time. Two years later to this day, she has yet to use her program. Her excuse is a familiar one: she doesn't have time right now to do it. I told her, "Look, the world will never give us a twenty-fifth hour in the day, so you might as well stop aspiring to have more time." She replied with, "You're right, I'll start next Monday." Yeah right! With two teen-aged kids and a husband who works full time and travels a lot, the household responsibilities all fall on her shoulders. However, I don't understand why she doesn't have time when she has two housekeepers who work eight hours a day for her. The problem is that food is her comfort so I believe she won't give that up. I also know that driving to the clinic in LA traffic held her back, too.

The first action step is to acquire better time-management skills, which will free up your mind and allow you to focus on your goals. When your behaviors become healthier, time suddenly frees up for healthy activities.

Some people who have mounds of mental clutter may need more than a self-help book. They might consider seeing a therapist to help sort through their mental clutter. Through therapy, a person may learn to develop objectivity when life gets tough. Choosing the right therapist can help you through life's toughest situations. Your family and friends might mean well, but sometimes their advice is ineffective and not objective. This can cause you to become anxious and feel alone and potentially helpless. This feeling leads you to the comfort zone that you know never fails you—food. But this choice will never solve anything in the long run, even if you feel safe in the moment.

You may be afraid to see a therapist. That feeling is normal. Seeing a therapist is only a suggestion. Regardless, once your life is in order, you'll lose weight. Start off by making to-do lists each day and meditating. Organize your mind, and life will feel better.

EXERCISES

(1) What is my to-do-list for the day?

(2) What healthy behaviors can I include?

(3) What is one piece of mind clutter that I have the ability to dump within the next week?

(4) What is my action plan for dumping this clutter?

TOOL 2. UNCLUTTER YOUR HOME

If your house is a mess, then your thoughts will also be a mess. Your house makes silent statements about how you feel about life. For you, it might feel comfortable just because you're used to it. You may also be used to being overweight, too, right? This doesn't mean you like it, and it doesn't mean that it's your life forever.

Go through each room in detail and decide if your home feels too comfortable. A cluttered home will make your weight-loss journey challenging. The comfort is no longer acceptable. Do what I used to do as the assistant general manager for The Sports Club/LA (now owned by Equinox.) I walked through the entire 130,000-square-foot club every day as if I were a potential member. My goal was to facilitate a jaw-dropping experience for every person who walked through the doors, as well as for the current members. I wanted our club to be a palace so that our members felt like royalty. To achieve this, I looked at the fine details of the club, including the condition of the walls, floors, counters, corners, ceilings, and everything in between. I documented everything and went back to each department head manager. I held them all accountable for fixing it.

Do this with your home. Relive your experience the first day you entered your home. Here's the assignment: walk through your front door as though you're entering your home for the very first time. Do you remember how much you loved your home back then? It was new. It was the perfect nest. Let's find that feeling again. Think about inviting someone over that you'd normally clean your house up for. Identify the specific things that need a tune-up. Have a pad and pen out and start writing those things down.

You can delegate tasks using your to-do list. Delegate these tasks to family members, or hire a personal assistant on Craigslist. They charge about twelve dollars an hour. A third alternative is to hire a teenaged neighbor who can always use the extra cash. Once your home is in order, life's daily commitments will suddenly appear so much easier for you because there's no more clutter to mess up your head. A cluttered head is one that picks the fork up and never puts it down.

In tool 65, we will discuss cleaning out your kitchen pantry and refrigerator.

EXERCISES

(1) What things in my home need to be fixed? (Make a list.)

(2) What is a realistic time frame for completion?

(3) Who is on my team to help me organize my home?

(4) Which rooms are my top priorities? (List the rooms in order of priority.)

TOOL 3. UNCLUTTER YOUR CAR

Personally, I can't stand it when my car has trash on the floor, bird droppings on the roof, empty water bottles on the floor, or used tissues and gum wrappers in the door pockets. It makes me feel like my car is a dumpster. Dumpsters accumulate trash. You must not accumulate trash in your car. A clean car also doesn't reek of burgers and stale fries. Gross! When your car is clean, you think clean. This will help translate into healthy eating.

Just think: a clean car can dissuade you from opening up a bag of messy potato chips or eating anything else that creates a mess. It would be quite annoying to eat junk food in a clean car because that would require many additional cleanups. Rather than mess it up, you'll most likely avoid it altogether, which removes another opportunity that allows for poor eating. Natural foods don't have horrific odors like junk food does. Mother Nature blends sweet aromas that put your mind at ease when you go fresh and healthy. Freshness from herbs, fruit, and vegetables give you an innate connection to Mother Nature. This fresh feeling of newness is like a brand-new car. Don't you love the smell and feeling of driving a new car? You feel good about yourself, and your sense of worth creates positive thoughts for your day. This is why you deserve to enter a new car that isn't polluted with clutter.

No matter what type of car it is, if it's clean, you'll feel worthy. Get it detailed. Get a car wash, vacuum it, clean out the trunk, organize the glove compartment, put a book in a seat pocket, clean out the trash, and add to the luxury.

In my experience with people I train, I have learned that more people than not who have weight issues also have cluttered cars. Cluttered cars are completely chaotic, and you never know where anything is. You don't even know where to start looking. You even justify your mess to others who drive with you. I never understood this. Why justify a habit that you know you can't stand?

Clean up your car and clean up your body! Both means of transportation get you around each day. Don't burn those motors out. Feed them with the right gas. Just like you put high-octane gas in your car, fuel your body's engine with vegetables, fruit, lean protein, nuts, seeds, and anything else that Mother Nature produces. If your vehicle has a trunk full of luggage, then you'll use more gas. If you're carrying extra weight around each day, then you'll waste more energy every day. This is why you feel like your body is always dragging. This is why you're exhausted, bloated, moody, and not performing at your best. Just as you drive your car without braking abruptly and killing the shocks, keep your muscles and joints healthy through the right type of exercise each week. In addition, it's imperative that you keep your body clear from any unnecessary stress and from genetically modified chemicals found in junk food, just like you keep your car clean from crumbs and clutter.

A clean car should symbolize your ability to rejoice in a body that's full of vitality so that in the end, you don't mind the work. You're rewarded by feeling loads of energy and eventually by receiving compliments from external sources.

EXERCISES

(1) What old habits do I plan on banning from my car?

(2) When will I give my car a makeover?

TOOL 4. UNCLUTTER YOUR WORKSPACE

Your workspace is a true reflection of how your mind operates. To be successful, you must keep an organized workspace that doesn't have any blemishes. Your workspace should have clean counters, a keyboard without food crumbs between the keys, a mouse pad without last week's food stains on it, and a dust-free desk. Keep your work-space clean by eating your meals away from your computer, which is more advantageous anyway. Eating away from your computer forces you to focus on the behavior of eating and nothing else. When you're unfocused, you eat more and you eat faster. When you eat faster, you don't thoroughly chew your food, and the right portion never satiates you.

Taking time to eat requires discipline. You might ask, "What if I'm too busy to eat away from my desk?" My response is to get your boss involved. Do you know that you'll be far more effective at task completion in the afternoon and you'll also lose weight? If you *are* the boss, then you need to showcase these behaviors to your employees by taking a break yourself. If they see you taking a formal break, then they will, too.

Employees who take lunch breaks are far more productive in their jobs compared to those who don't. A lunch break refreshes your mind and recharges you for the rest of your day. This increases productivity. Productive employees actually strengthen the company's bottom line. If you're in charge of your company, then I'm sure this is music to your ears.

We are a "cluttered mind" society that attempts to do everything all in one day. Not only is this impossible, but it also causes the quality of work to decline, which in turn causes tasks to take longer to complete. What a waste of money! Every employee should use a lunch period to unwind, debrief, and eat. Better mental acuity brings higher job satisfaction and higher employee retention rates. When an employee leaves a company, it's quite expensive to replace that employee. Keep them happy.

A lunch break will also reduce the number of times that you and your colleagues run to the candy jar at three p.m. for sugar to recharge. Sugar highs cause weight gain. Do you see a pattern? Let's break these poor behaviors by forming new habits that allow you to lose weight. Start a new health kick and help unclutter the whole office. Get everyone involved in becoming healthier by being the leader (tool 100).

The office should consider purchasing a refrigerator and kitchenette to encourage employees to eat away from their workstations. A refrigerator will also encourage people to pack healthy meals to bring to work. Rather than eating fast food or skipping meals, employees will eat better if they are given the appropriate environment. It wouldn't hurt to also throw in a water dispenser, especially since I'm a big fan of water consumption.

EXERCISES

(1) What part of my workspace resembles clutter?

(2) Where can I eat my lunch at work?

(3) What did I bring to work for lunch and snacks today?

(4) What is my action plan for incorporating a more organized lunch?

The art of uncluttering is a dynamic process and should be ongoing. Start believing in yourself. Have fun with this entire journey. Start appreciating the journey of change and the lessons you learn along the way. An open mind allows new information in. Push out the clutter that doesn't serve you and allow fun and good health to enter into your life.

Chapter 2

THE POWER OF YOUR MIND

Your mind is more powerful than you can even imagine. Therefore, stop ignoring it! Start embracing the act of feeding your mind with healthier outlets that will help you to cut back on stress and remain in an uncluttered state. It's time for you to fuel your own mind with tools that stimulate your personal potential. Having a powerful mind will give you the strength to turn away from food and turn toward healthier outlets that offer you mental satisfaction the way food used to.

TOOL 5. PRACTICE PATIENCE

To be lean, you must be patient, persistent, and perseverant. Be patient because it takes time, persistent because you shouldn't quit, and perseverant because you'll find unexpected challenges along the way. Patience can be a challenge for anyone with any goal, not just a weight-loss goal.

Many of you have done the weight loss thing many times in the past. Most of you have succeeded at losing weight but then put it right back on. It's time to really learn the ropes of losing weight once and for all. Let me ask you this; is it more important to have comfort food to save each day, or will you choose to save each year with physical activity and healthy food? I know most of you have said, "This diet sucks and doesn't work!" or "I should've lost at least twenty pounds by now and I haven't lost anything." This self-talk is very common among *dieters*. That's why you must stop calling your journey a *diet*. The sooner you stop calling it a diet, the sooner you'll accept the challenges along the way. You'll exercise because you want to. You'll eat healthier because you want to. Being patient with this process will allow you to get over your false expectations of change. You'll embrace the lifestyle that being healthy actually is, because you want to.

Unfortunately there's no quick-fix weight-loss pill out there that takes your weight off with the click of your heels. You must, therefore, start setting realistic goals for yourself. Stop trying to lose twenty pounds in a month. I promise you that quick weight loss is a loss of muscle versus fat anyway. This journey will differ from person to person, gender to gender, and race to race. Adopt a new mindset that embodies patience so that you never feel disappointed.

Weight loss is also unpredictable. People ask me when they'll hit their goal, but I'm not a psychic so I can't tell you. For example, I have a male client who lost twelve pounds in three weeks and a female client who's three years older than he is who lost three pounds in three weeks. Should she be upset? You might be nodding, but she shouldn't be. It's like comparing apples to oranges. The goal isn't how quickly you can lose weight but whether you can keep it off forever. I'd prefer slower weight loss because your body will lose fat and not muscle. Starvation diets result in severe atrophy. Atrophy is when your body loses muscle. Your body never uses fat when it starves. I'll never forget the time I handed a patient her credit card back and didn't sell her another weight-loss program. I told her, "Take your money and join the gym. You have no more weight to lose. It's time to lose your fat and tone up." She couldn't stop thanking me.

Dieters "yo-yo" and never master proper nutrition. Weight-loss students master healthier lifestyle habits. There's no such thing as perfect, so stop striving for perfection. If you eat a cookie, then suck it up and eat well at your next meal. Or, don't eat the cookie to begin with. It's seriously that easy. Motivating yourself from meal to meal is the key to success. Take any *poisonous* thoughts that bring your motivation down and toss them to the curb. Learning to be conscious is a form of practicing patience. Taking inventory of what's going on in your life allows things to change. The change that you open yourself up to will be the change that allows you to lose weight. When you play into the frustrations of not attaining your goal quickly enough, your motivation to change goes down the tubes. As a lean individual, my patience with myself is what keeps me lean and healthy. I translate this level of patience and consciousness into the areas of my life that require me to be more patient. I cannot tell you how effective this is. It's all about being open and honest with the process. This will bring change once you've mastered patience.

I can only spark the fire within you. The rest is up to you! Consider the things that might be holding you back from losing weight and where you can improve. Ask yourself each day the following questions and work on the things that need attention.

EXERCISES

(1) What motivates me to stay focused in this weight-loss journey?

(2) What is holding me back?

(3) How can I master patience today?

(4) What are the things I did right today? (Make a list.)

TOOL 6. PRACTICE YOGA

Yoga has been around for centuries and is known to re-center your core being while giving you access to your inner light. Your inner light can be compared to a flashlight that lights the path ahead of you when you're in the dark. Breath by breath you fuel your mind and body with new energy that provides you with endless potential for change. Your breath calms your nervous system down and puts you in a complete state of relaxation. Moving your breath through your body allows you to clear your muscles, joints and your mind from toxic clutter that causes you poor health. During your weight-loss journey, you must be balanced and have a clear mind for the things that need to change. If your body is tight, your mind will not be balanced. Yoga can ground you and allow you to be in tune with your body on a deeper level. Chronic stress and disconnect will impede this ability.

Certain postures in yoga class may feel awkward. Stay committed and allow yourself the chance to embody a new practice. Time and practice will make you better. The great thing about yoga is that it's a practice. The more you practice the better you get. Start with a beginner level one class. There are many out there. You may even consider taking a restorative class, which includes passive stretching and breathing exercises, as your introduction to yoga. Yoga offers the following benefits:

- Yoga invites you to listen to your body.

- Yoga decreases discomfort in your mind and body.

- Yoga teaches you proper breathing.

- Yoga works on muscle strength, endurance, and flexibility through movements that rid your body of toxins from the day.

- Yoga helps achieve a state of relaxation and meditation.

- Yoga improves circulation to all the vital organs.

- Yoga creates a sound mind.

- Yoga helps you with spiritual realization.

- Yoga helps you fall in love with yourself.

- Yoga releases bad energy.

- Yoga helps reduce tension and pain.

- Yoga teaches you how to be fearless.

- Yoga helps you open your heart up to the world.

I understand that yoga can appear slow at first for some and very hard for others. The great news is, you get to work within your own level of comfort without any judgments or failure involved.

Allow a yoga class to clear your mind. Work through the tension in your body and offer your body freedom from your *chains*. Feel good in your own skin. In fact, you should feel amazing in your own skin. Be limber both mentally and physically so that calmness clears the way for healthier actions. No matter how much you weigh, there are plenty of yoga moves that'll allow you to accomplish a euphoric feeling after taking a class.

Some people experience discomfort during class. If you have a legitimate injury, then certain classes may not be right for you. If you don't have an injury, then you need to tweak your practice. Ask your instructor for alternative poses prior to the class. Many classes and teachers offer modified positions or yoga tools such as a block or a strap to help people with less flexibility or with minor injuries.

If you want to do yoga at home, then count on my teacher, Tamal Dodge, (www.tamalyoga.com) or www.corepoweryoga.com for great yoga DVD workouts. You can also find yoga teachers in your area who will do a one-hour session in the privacy of your own home.

Practicing yoga allows you to appreciate your body and your life. You'll eventually want to treat your body like gold. Eating refined carbohydrates, sugar, or fried foods is treating your body like a garbage bin. Bring organic ways into your day. Unclutter your mind and reignite your inner light. Namaste!

EXERCISES

(1) Where is the closest yoga studio to me?

(2) What are five yoga poses I can do each day?

TOOL 7. MEDITATE

Many people tell me that they've tried meditation on multiple occasions and have failed to arrive at a true still point in their minds. I find it hard to believe that these individuals have had a true meditation experience if this is the case. People have so much going on in their heads that they'll simply plop themselves down somewhere, close their eyes, and start thinking about what they're thinking about. That's not meditation, and it won't relax you.

I recently met with a patient whose primary doctor told him he is hypertensive and that he needs blood pressure medication immediately. This sent him into a panic. I told him that he needed to calm his very stressful life down. He was striving to be number one out of over six thousand other employees in his company nationwide. Always being number one meant always cluttering his mind every single year. His body was crying for help. High blood pressure was only one indication.

I laid him down on a yoga mat and took him through a breathing exercise that focused on deep pelvic breathing and meditation. Three minutes into the exercise, he opened up his eyes and asked me, "Are we almost done?" I thought to myself, "Oy vey!" He is a great example of someone who is consumed with work beyond my ability to help him. His mind will always race, and his heart and body will eventually deteriorate if he doesn't recognize the need to change.

Meditation is the art of self–involvement that aligns your energy with that of the universe. Meditation is the ability to remove your conscious thoughts from reality and escape into the land of calmness and serenity. You can achieve this in Shavasana during yoga practice.

If you're like how I used to be and your mind is moving at the speed of light every second of the day, then meditation is exactly what you need. I used to over-commit myself to the world, which caused me to live outside of my body. I got sick more often, experienced fatigue, and would be unexpectedly moody. I had to consciously change this by introducing yoga classes, meditation, and even acupuncture and chiropractic into my life. Sleep is another area that I've improved over the years. You must calm your body and mind so that you can handle life's stressful situations more effectively. Calming your body and mind will also facilitate weight loss. Meditation is an art that unclutters your mind (tool 1). You owe this to your body.

You must first want to engage in meditation practices. Knowing and doing are two different things. As preposterous as it might sound, all of us have a still point within us. Learning how to incorporate patience into your practice allows for a place of mental stillness. It isn't easy the first few times, which is why many people give up after attempting it on a superficial level.

If getting to a meditative state is challenging for you, then consider hiring a professional to help get you started. If you don't know where to start, then seek out an alternative healer. There are other disciplines, such as Reiki, acupuncture, yoga retreats, some chiropractic treatment centers, and some massage therapists who can help you get there. Each of these disciplines facilitates mental and physical calmness. Look in your local area for the professionals who offer these innovative self-discovery opportunities. There are also many meditation CDs available. Once you start looking, you'll be amazed at how many resources are available to you right in your own backyard.

EXERCISES

(1) Do my friends know of any great alternative practitioners?

(2) What is my goal for meditating today?

(3) Who can help me do the Ferris wheel exercise? (Do the Ferris wheel exercise with someone who can help you create your still point. Have them read you the following sample exercise. When someone else reads it, you can focus on the words and fall into meditation.)

Close your eyes. Picture a Ferris wheel. Do you know the gigantic, illuminated circular device at theme parks? Well, let's pretend that the Ferris wheel never stops. Draw your attention from the perimeter of the wheel, where all the blinking lights are, and follow the spokes toward the center of the wheel, where all the spokes meet. If you look into the very center, you can still see movement, but you'll notice that the movement gets much smaller and more precise compared to the movement on the outer edges of the Ferris wheel. Imagine going deeper into the spokes of the wheel beyond the metal, in through the paint, and through the very center of the Ferris wheel. Then, keep going in deeper, and you will eventually not see any form of movement at the core of the wheel. We can call that point the still point. It's so deep, that movement isn't seen by the naked eye. Bring your focus to that still point. Acknowledge the center as the place where all movement stems from. The moving parts of the Ferris wheel meet at a place of stillness. Bring your body to that place of stillness. Allow your center to be your still point. Inhale into that space. Exhale out of that space. Inhale with newfound energy; exhale any stagnant energy. Allow the breath to be your source of movement while maintaining a still point in your mind. Inhale through the nose and exhale through the nose and back of your throat to create the sound of ocean waves kissing the shore. In yoga, we call this the ujjayi breath. Keep breathing. Steady breaths, just relax.

TOOL 8. LIGHT A CANDLE

Think about your daily behaviors when you run out the door in the morning. You go through your workday with lots of pressure and stress. You drive in horrible traffic past terrible drivers and feel overwhelmed because, as usual, you're running late. You're running here and there-it's just exhausting! This may not be your exact story, but the American story is generally a chaotic one. The human body is *not* built for this, yet you continue doing this every single day. You're the only one who can stop this pattern for yourself.

A candle symbolizes many different things in our lives. It can represent the little fire in your heart that reminds you to remain motivated every day. The light can also allow your heart to open up to the light of good health and positive energy. If coming home at night brings you personal chaos, then you'll be exhausted and unmotivated to work on yourself. This chaotic lifestyle causes stress that can make you sick. You must therefore adopt relaxation tools such as lighting a candle and even listening to calming music.

Take a moment when you get home. Pause and light your favorite scented candle such as lavender, sage, rosemary, or lemon. These scents will calm your mind down and help ease tension. Other scents are okay as long as they calm you down and allow you to take control of your evening. Let the little light burn in front of you as you cook up a healthy dinner for yourself and your family. Allow that candle to burn as you help your children with their homework. Let the light burn while you listen to your spouse's day, look through your mail, practice yoga, or do whatever you do when you get home.

The central light will remind you of the calm place inside of you that contains positive and loving energy for yourself. It's good to feel safe in your own home. Relaxation comes from lighting a candle because it gives you a sense of centeredness, which is calming.

Take the imagery of that candle's fire and ignite your own internal flame of motivation. Rather than allowing your flame to burn viciously within you, and possibly overwhelm you, learn how to control it to the appropriate height so that it's just enough to make you feel content and inspired to make the necessary changes in your lifestyle. You will feel more in control of your life. Your actions will be more calm and concise. Calming your mind down after a long day will also allow the pieces of your day to fall into place more naturally and not forcefully. This is an excellent formula for healthy aging, too.

EXERCISES

(1) Where in my home can I put candles to help facilitate serenity?

(2) Other than a candle, what are two other tools I can use to bring calmness into my home after a long day's work?

TOOL 9. RENT A RELAXING MOVIE

Ongoing stress takes a terrible toll on your body. It increases inflammation and inhibits your ability to cope with more stress. Inflammation leads to *zero* weight loss. When you're calm, you're more logical and you release fewer stress hormones (cortisol is the worst), which will improve your ability to lose weight. Chronic stress throws off virtually everything in your body including your blood pressure, gastrointestinal health, hormones, adrenal glands, musculoskeletal systems, cholesterol, and other systems.

When you're experiencing stressful patches in your life, relaxation is crucial. Stress release can be achieved by escaping into the world of cinema. Exercise can definitely be another outlet, but sometimes your body simply needs rest. (Sometimes—not always!) Companies like RedBox have vending machines that rent movies for only a dollar and change. I know a lot of people who have either a Netflix or Hulu account. There are other ways to score a movie. The goal is to get one and then relax.

Once in a while I'll rent a total chick flick when I'm alone. My favorite movie of all time is *Can't Buy Me Love*. I still can't get over how Patrick Dempsey evolved from that dorky little lawn-mower guy. When I was a little girl, I aspired to be like Cynthia, who was the captain of the varsity cheerleaders in that movie. (Of course, in real life I had to make that happen.) Sometimes I rent a cartoon animation. I know—I'm like a kid. So? We all get to pick which movies lower our stress levels, right? Mentally dissolve yourself into a good movie. You will feel so much better afterward.

If you're dealing with sadness then it's best to consider renting a comedy. Laughter and smiling are the best medicines for everything. I always say that if I can make people laugh, then I've done a great deed—even if it's at my expense.

Take the night to unwind in the privacy of your own home or go to a movie theater. Invite a friend or ask your spouse or child to watch the movie with you. Make it a healthy night by snacking on a fistful of almonds with an apple or a cup of carrot and celery sticks with a quarter cup of hummus dip. Drink a bottle of water and make sure you're relaxed and not thinking about anything else but the movie.

There's nothing in life that's worth stressing about to the level that most people experience. We stress out simply because we're conditioned to. I'm talking about the stress that's a learned behavior. It's up to you to identify when you're overwhelmingly stressed and address these times by diving into a calming experience, like watching a movie. It's time to recognize when stress is overruling your existence and stop it before it gets worse.

EXERCISES

(1) Which stressors will I dismiss by renting a movie?

(2) What types of movies calm me down and put me in a great mood?

(3) What is the name of the last movie I watched, and when did I watch it?

(4) What movies would I like to see but haven't seen yet?

TOOL 10. DRAW A PICTURE

On Donald Trump's *Celebrity Apprentice* on April 3, 2011, the task was to create artwork on canvas and design hats and other art to raise as much money as possible at an auction. The team that sold the most artwork won the task. None of these celebrities were true artists, but they all appeared to be having fun. Art truly brings you peace and tranquility while dipping into your creative side.

You don't need to be another Pablo Picasso when you draw. Creating artwork enables you to feel good about yourself. It's quite rewarding to find something you like to draw such as a beautiful skyline, a mountain range with birds flying over it, cloud formations, a breathtaking sunset, palm trees against a watercolor sky, or an original design. Simply allow your creative juices to flow onto the canvas or sketchpad, and watch yourself incorporate a whole new calmness into your day. Draw the room you're sitting in, the dream you had last night, or the image of the world you wish to live in.

When I was in high school, I took an art class and painted our backyard as the leaves changed colors heading into fall. I remember sitting on one of the steps next to the driveway and looking off into a sea of colors. Although it caused me to procrastinate from my studies, it relaxed me after a busy day.

Drawing puts the right cerebral hemisphere to work, too. The right part of your brain contains your imaginative sense, your intuition, your visual center, and it also controls your state of consciousness. Weight-loss success stems from your being in the conscious state of mind so that you make the right decisions. Doesn't it make sense to wake this part of the brain up?

It's very likely that your community offers art classes. Art class teaches you how to live in a state of consciousness through observation and attention to detail. Creativity links your ability to trust your own intuition as well. Most of the time, your gut instinct won't steer you wrong. Because drawing is a self-involved activity, you're forced to be in tune with yourself on a deeper level than ever before. This oneness can easily extend to other areas of your life where you need it the most. Allow this power to stimulate your vision of a very successful weight-loss journey.

EXERCISES

(1) What will I draw?

(2) Do I need lessons?

(3) What medium will I use (e.g., canvas, paper, a wall)?

TOOL 11. READ A BOOK

Reading opens up your mind to new information. Mental fitness is part of this journey, too. Reading more information about your goal creates a clear pathway so you can actively become part of the solution.

Whenever I want to learn something new, I conduct my own research on the topic and self-educate before going to the experts. The information sinks in more effectively when you do this. Turning to the experts for all the answers and never attempting to learn something on your own, may impede your ability to effectively process the information.

Reading jogs your memory, stimulates your mind, and expands your imagination. For some, it offers a better vocabulary. There are books on how to conquer specific fitness goals, how to cut down debt, how to learn a new craft, how to understand basic law, how to develop more self-love, and a host of other topics that may interest you. Go to the bookstore and explore.

Dive into a novel, love story, or even a mystery book. Tickle your imagination to help unfold the neurological pathways for better mental acuity. Find a bedside book, a bathroom book, and a waiting room book. Incorporate books into your everyday life. Always keep your mind stimulated so that you can keep your organs functioning at optimal levels throughout your life. A healthy mind tops a healthy body. Mental stimulation may retard the early onset of brain diseases such as Alzheimer's. I have noticed that brain health declines in people who retire and no longer have to utilize their brains for complex matters. Don't let this be you: keep that mind running.

EXERCISES

(1) What am I interested in learning?

(2) Which book will I read next?

(3) How many books would I like to read each month?

TOOL 12. RESCUE AN ANIMAL

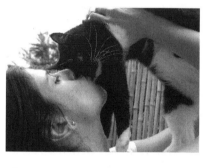

Some women say to me, "Yeah, I rescued an animal all right. I married my husband!" Funny, right? All jokes aside, rescuing an animal opens up a whole new world of opportunity for you to be more active while calming your stress levels down. Pets offer friendship as well as positive energy after a long grueling day.

Dogs require you to walk them, which helps increase your daily movement. The bigger the dog, the bigger the workout. You'll have to control it by using muscular force to control your new curious friend from intimidating other pedestrians. You'll also need to move briskly to keep up with it. You can also rescue a small dog. Small dogs still require you to walk them but require much less muscular work than big dogs do. It makes me sad when I go to someone's house and he or she fails to walk the dog. I know people who simply open up their back door and allow their dog to do its thing right in the backyard. (Be cautious in people's yards these days. Yeah—gross!) Dogs need movement just as much as we do. If you get a dog then don't neglect it. Take it on a morning and evening walk. Choose a power walk so you can elevate your heart rate while your dog gets cardiovascular exercise, too.

Perform intervals with your dog so you can burn more calories and fat. For example, bring a stick or a ball with you. Toss the object far and make your dog run after it. Run after your dog. Repeat this five times, and then recover for five minutes by simply walking. After you recover your energy, repeat the interval set again. Work your way up to a second interval set if you can't achieve it initially. Remember, Rome wasn't built in a day, so neither is your fitness level.

Walking a minimum of twenty minutes a day will help you so much. Elevating your heart rate through intervals will help you burn fat and calories. Warm up prior to going on this walk so you don't pull a muscle.

For those of you who don't want the huge responsibility of a dog, there are cats. Just know that cats must be played with and stimulated each day to keep them young and illness free. Even though cats are independent, they still demand love and attention. You can play chase with them for twenty minutes a day. My cat, Bebe, is very active and demands daily playtime with me. She's athletic and brings such joy into my life. I wrestle with her on the floor and run through the house using the laser light and cat toy on a wire. Don't think I'm crazy, but we also play hide-and-seek. When I catch her, she sprawls out on the floor. I perform ten really slow push-ups and kiss her belly in between reps. This gets me to move more and stretch each night while working.

Consider an animal a friend that offers you a synergistic relationship: both of you benefit from having each other. Animals can also help lower your stress levels, too. They give you unconditional love as long as you feed them and clean up after them.

EXERCISES

(1) Which pet do I own or wish to own?

(2) If I already have a pet, how will I add more play time into our day together?

TOOL 13. WELCOME THE CHANGE

Change is hard to undergo. However, it reinvents who we are as people. How we embrace change is a strong indication of our true character. You can choose to be strong through saying, "I welcome change wherever change is necessary!" Losing weight requires change in some of the things you do. Start asking yourself, "What is hindering my weight-loss success, and what needs to change?" Think consciously. Be excited about the change. You actually begin to enjoy life so much more when you welcome change. With your nutritional goals, make the conscious decision to stop blaming "the diet" for not achieving your goal soon enough. Embrace the barriers that are in the way of attaining your weight-loss goal, and then learn to treat this journey as a *lifestyle*.

Some people tell me that their love for sweets and salt is a hard barrier to overcome. Cravings can be a challenge. The great news is that there are healthy alternatives out there such as nuts, carrot sticks dipped in hummus, french-cut green beans, cucumber slices topped with light Laughing Cow cheese, and low-fat cottage cheese parfait topped with walnuts and berries, to name a few. Cravings also stem from your lack of eating *small frequent meals* (tool 31) throughout the day like you're supposed to. Start eating small portions frequently and you won't find yourself binging at night. Nighttime eating is the worst. Learn how much protein you should eat each day before you proceed (tool 59). To start, I am a big advocate for cutting out all high glycemic carbohydrates for at least four weeks. I understand that some people get deterred from following these strict guidelines. However, when you cut out the bread, pasta, rice, potatoes and sweets, you are left with food that your body *needs* versus *wants*. Your body needs fruits and vegetables, but most likely doesn't get enough of those food groups. When you eliminate all of the high glycemic carbohydrates, you begin to see results in all areas of your life; mentally, physically, and emotionally. It is worth the big jump because in the end, you feel better. As aggressive as this approach may appear, it works well to help lower cravings for the foods that also cause your blood sugar to spike.

Accepting the change means adopting the characteristics of who you want to be. This book is exposing you to the lifestyle habits of a lean individual. Find enjoyment in these new lifestyle decisions. Both you and I know that you don't like being overweight. Being lean and healthy means accepting the fact that you can't just drive up to a fast-food restaurant when you're in a hurry. Being lean and healthy means not popping candy into your mouth because you have cravings. Your lifestyle behaviors must change so that you can change your weight. Be prepared each day with the right combinations, and you will feel like a million bucks. Oh, and you'll lose weight, too.

EXERCISES

(1) Do I fear change?

(2) Which change is hard for me? Why?

(3) How will the changes I make be rewarded? (Food should not be used.)

TOOL 14. STOP SPENDING SPARE TIME WITH OVERWEIGHT PEOPLE

Ever hear the expression, "You are who you hang out with?" I'm not putting overweight people down, so please forgive me for bluntly saying this. The number one complaint I hear from people trying to lose weight is "Everybody always tries to sabotage me and I keep falling off track!" I'm sure that many of you have been victims to saboteurs. When I ask dieters who these people are, they're usually family members, friends, colleagues, or spouses. Ninety-nine percent of the time (my own statistic) they are overweight themselves. Furthermore, surrounding your-self with poor behaviors will unmotivate you to make any changes yourself. Most overweight company will sit, eat, and talk rather than go hiking, teach you a new healthy recipe, take a yoga class with you, or do something to pro-mote good health. Dining out with overweight people may also expose you to suboptimal restaurants that don't have many healthy options to choose from. In addition, the peer pressure to eat poorly is always a factor in this scenario. Being lean requires you to be different from others in this type of group. I've been told that there's social awkward-ness when you're the only one who modifies the menu while everyone else simply chooses right from it. I've also been told that it's tiresome to have to think about what's acceptable to eat after working a long week. People don't even like the attention that healthy eating brings them. Many of their friends don't even support their journey. So hang out with healthier people. Your journey will be far more successful when you hang out with a fit crowd.

The alternative is to hang out with people you want to and just eat healthily regardless of how they eat. Always order dressings and sauces on the side, keep fried food completely out of your vocabulary, steam the vegetables, and ditch the bread and any other high-glycemic carbohydrates (tool 68). Drink plenty of water with your meal even if others drink diet soda (aspartame—yuck!) or regular soda (far too much sugar). When people order a soda when they're with me, it always makes me laugh when they look over at me for my approval. I simply shrug my shoulders as if to say, "It's your body, not mine!" Surrounding yourself with healthy people makes losing weight easier.

EXERCISES

(1) Whom do I eat with?

(2) Are there any saboteurs in my weight-loss journey?

(3) What changes will I apply to my life today?

TOOL 15. ACKNOWLEDGE YOUR FOOD ADDICTION

You may very well have a physiological and neurological dependence on food that must be broken. Many people do. The only way to break your addiction is to stop eating the items that cause the addiction. In modern-day society, food is often used as a drug to satisfy sadness, depression, stress, and boredom. When food is used to fill a mental void, it eventually becomes an addictive substance. Out of the many researchers out there, I was attracted to the work done by Dr. Robert Pretlow. He conducted a very interesting study involving children who demonstrated signs of addiction to food. His 2010 prospective analysis viewed 134,000 messages that were posted in an online chat room. The chat room hosted conversations between obese children communicating the effects they felt from eating. His analysis revealed that kids described their pleasurable relationship with food in a way that satisfied nearly all the DSM-IV addiction criteria. The DSM-IV is considered the bible for psychologists to aid them in determining any and all mental disorders in their patients. Dr. Pretlow outlined how children turned their emotional desire for food into a neurological dependency over time. He blamed the dopamine receptors in the brain since he found similarities between the dopamine levels in obese individuals and the dopamine levels in drug-addicted individuals. Remember, dopamine is the neurotransmitter that is responsible for reward and pleasure in the brain. Once these receptors experience cravings at the receptor sites, there is now a neurological addiction to that substance. This study will open up new avenues for research in the future.

This is serious stuff. Food has turned into an abused substance for both adults and children due to high levels of stress. The bad news is that food is a required substance to sustain life. But if people are using food for anything other than survival, then the food addiction will continue to live. For some, medical supervision is needed to help break the food addiction. Recognizing that you have an addiction is the first step. Breaking the addiction through intervention is the next step.

Consider doing a cleanse (tool 37) to break your addiction. On a cleanse, you eat a lot of vegetables and fruits for seven days. This will help change your palate and you will begin to crave natural foods when you finish. Bringing your blood sugars back to normal levels after the cleanse will diminish your cravings for sugar and allow you to stick to low glycemic (tool 68) eating. This will make your weight loss journey much easier and ultimately successful.

Learn self-control and portion control. Your choices and portions of food will determine your weight loss success. Keep a food journal (tool 28). I know you may love fast food and high-glycemic carbohydrates. Just remember, high-glycemic carbohydrates spike your blood sugar level, causing mega doses of insulin to secrete from your pancreas. Just get rid of *all* high glycemic carbohydrates (see tool 68) for four weeks, and you will learn that your body doesn't *need* them.

Here are two patients whose stories ended on a positive note:

1) The first patient had a midnight habit of consuming an entire can of whipped cream. She was addicted to sugar and chose whipped cream to satisfy her sugar craving because it was *low fat*. She would spray an entire can of whipped cream down her throat and go to the grocery store at midnight to buy more if necessary. She was twenty pounds overweight and couldn't lose a pound. The good news is that she was able to acknowledge that this wasn't okay, and she sought help.

   How did she kick this habit? First she identified the things in her life that caused her to do this. She hated her job. Her boss was harassing her and lowering her self-esteem. This caused her to go home every day feeling depressed. She found comfort in eating crackers and cheese and other foods that weren't nutritious. This led her to consume whipped cream an hour later due to a sugar low right before bedtime. These eating patterns caused her to sleep poorly. She woke up groggy every morning and felt even more depressed the next day. After hearing about her day, I asked her if she realized that she was addicted to food. She said she did.

As you now know, when you turn to any substance for emotional comfort to help guard you from stress, it can turn into an addiction. In her case, food was her substance abuse. She addressed her emotional distress and learned how to treat food as a source of survival, not as a source for comfort. To this day, she's successfully maintaining her lean body weight and is working at a different company. It took her time, but she did it. This change allowed her to find love for herself again.

2) Another client, who is a physician, worked odd hours and turned to candy to get through her long days. She used her lack of time as an excuse to eat poorly while at work. Her candy addiction carried over into the evening, when she consumed an entire box of low-fat ice cream bars. She did this every night. She wasn't losing weight. Anyone know why? Her days were filled with high-glycemic carbohydrates, which caused nighttime cravings. This was her first problem. Sugar was her drug, which caused

her blood sugar levels to spike high and drop low all throughout the day.

We identified three major problems that drove these behaviors: (1) she wasn't getting enough quality sleep each night; (2) she was battling minor depression due to boredom; and (3) she didn't go to work prepared to eat small, frequent meals each day. Small, frequent meals with the right macronutrient distribution would prevent the sugar spikes that exacerbated her cravings. She was able to acknowledge this. She started to journal and plan out her days. She changed her work schedule and no longer works many back-to-back night shifts anymore. This gave her time to shop for healthy food that she could bring to work. She now goes to bed at a reasonable hour each night and started taking Zumba classes, which added more joy to her week. Out of forty pounds, she lost twenty-five pounds in a six month period. She is well on her way.

Some of you may not have a sugar addiction, but you love bread and other high-glycemic carbohydrates such as fruit juice, crackers, bagels, cereal, or rice. These foods hinder weight loss, too. No matter what the food is, it's up to you to break your addiction. Breaking your addiction will help melt the pounds right off of you. Give yourself at least six months to a year. Healthy food consumption diminishes cravings. Remember, consistency is the key to your success. You will eventually break your addiction to food in time. Be patient with yourself, and don't hesitate to get help.

EXERCISES

(1) Which food am I addicted to?

(2) What kind of pleasure do I get when I eat this food?

(3) How long have I been addicted to food?

(4) What will I do to kick my food addiction?

TOOL 16. SAY "I CAN"

Some people go into a weight-loss program for the gazil-lionth time and plan on *failing* before they begin. These people have the distance between their ears to blame. Your thoughts can truly sabotage you, or they can work in your favor. Think "I can" and stop setting yourself up for failure. Have you ever studied for a test in school and said, "I'm totally gonna fail this test" and then you passed it? I doubt it.

Sabotaging thoughts create negative results. Let's parallel this to weight loss. Adopt the mindset of successful weight loss by believing in yourself. Don't make up your mind that you'll fail. Stop saying, "I'll try!" Part ways with any thoughts of failing. Don't make failing an option. You'll have many hiccups in the road even on this new path. How you deal with each hiccup will determine your success in the long run.

Tools to combat negativity include the following:

- Use the same *fire* that you possessed when you fought hard for your career, during college, for your children's success, and for any other endeavor you're proud of.

- Write down any negative thoughts that come to mind during weight loss and crumple that piece of paper up. Toss it into the trashcan where it belongs. Negative thinking never works.

- Identify the tools you'll need to proceed with your weight-loss journey.

- Flood your mind with positive affirmations and replace "I can't" or "I'll try" with "I can."

- Surround yourself with positive people and inspirational quotes.

Remember, there's no such thing as failing. You're the driver of your own ship. You can steer yourself successfully down the river of opportunity, or you can go against the river and battle upstream. Steering yourself down the river rather than up against the tide means learning from each hiccup you encounter and actually growing from it. The goal is to be well equipped to cope with future hiccups that cross your path again. Learning good strategies to help you overcome your difficulties in this journey makes you a stronger person. You'll gain mental perseverance.

In all the years I've been coaching people in weight loss, mental perseverance seems to be the missing link.

Remember, no one is perfect at anything in life. Don't strive for perfection when it comes to weight loss. You're a human being. Give yourself a chance to learn and grow from your hiccups. Find joy in your journey of personal growth. It's quite beautiful when you open your eyes up to it.

EXERCISES

(1) Which tools helped me succeed in other areas of life?

(2) What things have stopped me in the past from successfully losing weight?

(3) What needs to change in my life to help promote real weight loss?

(4) Have I said, "Yes, I can do it!" today?

TOOL 17. IDENTIFY YOUR MOMENT OF TRUTH

Your moment of truth is defined as your reflection of something that was said to you and impacted you in a memorable way, something great that happened to you, or something you witnessed someone else doing.

Moments of truth should focus on *what is* rather than what isn't. When you embrace moments in your day that bring you positive thoughts and feelings, you retain an internal glow, which helps you to walk away from unhappy thoughts. If being depressed, disappointed, and lonely causes you to eat poorly, then you should create a list of things that bring you out of the darkness and into the light. Paying close attention to the moments of truth throughout the day allows you to get out of the darkness.

Introduce moments of truth to business meetings, outings with friends, or during dinner with your family. First explain what moments of truth are. Then go around the room asking everyone to share their daily moment of truth. It actually increases your ability to bond with these individuals on a deeper level each day. It also enables everyone to practice public speaking. The conversation will have depth, and you will notice that when people share their truth, they actually feel good about telling their story.

Moments of truth are always positive. Even if your moment wasn't full of laughter, it should be something that ultimately helped you feel humbled and emotionally fulfilled for the day. A great example was when I was standing in line for the ATM machine and a young gentleman barged through the bank doors on his cell phone. However, when he entered the bank, he looked behind him to see a geriatric man limping toward the bank. Despite his hurry, he stopped everything in his world to hold the door for the limping man. He then proceeded to the counter to fill out his deposit slip, and the older gentleman limped over to thank him for his kindness. I got to witness this entire scenario. This was my moment of truth. I learn repeatedly that we must slow down and take a moment to see beautiful moments as such. Otherwise, you may miss helping someone who's in true need of your assistance.

Ditch any negative thoughts before you look for moments of truth. Take a moment now and simply relive your day in your head. Write down the series of events that happened today. Find the areas of joy and let them light up your day. We all have many.

Below are sample moments of truth that pertain to a person's weight loss journey:

- You went to the gym and met a very nice woman who is interested in your new business idea while you were working out on the elliptical. You realize now that you wouldn't have met her if you didn't go to the gym.

- You drank eighty ounces of water today because for the first time ever, you actually counted the bottles of water you drank. You also realized that your water intake allowed you to eat less calories for the day.

- You made the lunch-hour yoga class, which encouraged you to eat a very lean lunch afterward. You felt quite relaxed and refreshed, which is why you ate well.

Recognize your moments of truth every day. Share them with someone. This should be in your life for life. You deserve to feel a sense of accomplishment every day.

EXERCISES

(1) What was my biggest moment of truth today?

(2) How did this moment of truth affect me?

(3) Can I think of additional truths today? What are they?

TOOL 18. EAT JUNK FOOD TWICE A MONTH

Your body is the biggest creature of habit. Consistently eating well teaches it how to sustain normal daily blood sugar levels. When you "cheat" only twice a month, your body can handle it. Daily cheating disables the body from learning. Therefore, indulge in the foods you crave only two *designated days a month.* Self-control on all other days will allow you to attain your goal weight without a problem.

Take my example. I grew up in New York, and I would argue that New York has the best pizza and bagels in the world. I don't eat pizza or bagels regularly here in California simply because it doesn't compare to New York food in my opinion. My friend calls California the land of salads. Anyway, the three times a year I visit New York, I treat myself to whatever I want. I allow myself New York pizza and a bagel topped with cream cheese, lox, and whitefish salad. Do you know how many calories my days contain when I'm out there? I'll put it to you this way, if I ate that stuff every day and didn't live the way I do here in Los Angeles, I wouldn't have the credentials to teach you how to break your chains of obesity. My average stay in New York is four days. That would equal at most fifteen days a year that I eat poorly in New York. Altogether, I splurge approximately twenty-five to thirty times a year out of 365 days a year. Not too bad when you keep it in perspective. I splurge in New York, on my birthday (no calories ever count on your birthday), on Christmas, for New Years, on vacations (one per year), during the Fourth of July, on Memorial Day, on Labor Day, and maybe at an event here and there. My self-control helps me to behave this way without ever feeling guilty.

Schedule your junk-food days. Do you have any weddings, birthday parties, holidays, or anniversaries this month? Look at a calendar for the month and commit yourself ahead of time. Make sure those two days are filled with food that's worth the calories.

If you have a horrific sweet tooth, then these free days will exacerbate cravings for wanting more sweets or salt if you overdo it. Portion control is important. The more sugar you eat, the more your body will want it. If overindulging in sugar is part of your free day, then be prepared on a healthy day to combat cravings. You can be successful at this by exercising that day so that your body has a better chance at burning up the junk food you ate. You should also promise yourself not to feel guilty about enjoying your two junk-food days.

I should mention that many people fear free days during their weight-loss journey. I understand that the fear stems from not being able to get back on track once they go off for a day. This will only be a challenge if you allow it to be. Free days should only serve as a break from the high level of focus you possess in your journey. The goal behind a free day is to refrain from any frustrations you build up, allowing you to recharge your motivation battery.

Remember, two days a month *only*. Make sure you schedule them in advance, and stick to the schedule. Free days are not required; they are only an option to hold you sane through your transformation.

EXERCISES

(1) Which two days will be my free days this month?

(2) What are my fears about having two free days each month?

(3) What will my plan be to conquer my fears?

TOOL 19. DITCH THE ALCOHOL

Ask yourself if you even need to drink at all. Does it calm you down after a long workday? If that's the case and you don't want to completely ditch alcohol, then can you settle for one glass of wine? Men, don't drink more than two glasses a night. Women, stick to one glass. Chronic alcohol consumption stalls weight loss for everyone.

If you ditch the alcohol altogether, then losing weight will be easier. All alcohol possesses calories. Calorie restriction is crucial during weight loss. Although I'm not a big fan of counting calories, I do believe that being educated about the right foods for the best fuel is vital in your weight-loss journey. Consciously remind yourself that alcohol offers your body no nutritional benefit. Yes, I know that wine contains good stuff. However, the caloric cost compared to the benefits isn't worth it for a *loser*. Does this convince you to skip your nightcap?

Great story I wish to share: A patient didn't understand why he wasn't losing weight or body fat since he was eating well. I found out that he was drinking a bottle of wine every night. He insisted that he would not ditch the wine and told me that I should never bring it up to him again. I said, "Okay but I don't want *you* to bring up to me that you want to be 15 percent body fat—deal?" He agreed to this deal and has yet to hit his goal to this day. He actually increased his body fat over the course of the year, which is worse than gaining weight. I use him as an example because he was convinced that things would eventually work for him despite his wine drinking. He was wrong.

Weight plateaus are another interesting dynamic. Some people make the mistake of blaming an increase in muscle mass for the lack of weight loss when in reality it's most likely due to poor nutrition. If you're lifting very heavy weights and performing one to six repetitions for weeks at a time, eating a lot of protein, and taking certain supplements, then maybe. I doubt this is your story. The best way to verify this is to retest your total body composition (tool 50). Rather than rationalize your lack of progress, identify why you're not losing weight and simply adjust your behaviors accordingly. If drinking too much wine or other sugary libations is the problem, then change your habits to one glass per night. Then reassess. If you lack self-control, then find an alternative stress reliever other than food or alcohol.

Cigarette smoking isn't an alternative either. The cells in your body will be as healthy as you treat them. Toxic substances such as nicotine, alcohol, artificial sweeteners, and other chemicals seen in food are never the answer. You now have a whole book of tools to choose from. Take advantage of them!

I have seen so many people lose weight successfully once they took control of their emotions and thoughts. Alcohol ruins sleep, increases body fat, increases your triglyceride levels, and frustrates you in the end. It's just not worth it.

EXERCISES

(1) How many alcoholic drinks on average do I have a week?

(2) When and why do I usually drink?

(3) What alternative stress relievers will I experiment with so I can ditch the alcohol?

TOOL 20. CONFIDE IN SOMEONE YOU TRUST

This tool deals with the art of uncluttering as I discussed in tools 1–4. If you're overwhelmed with something stressful from your past or your present, then you should learn how to debrief. Debriefing is having a conversation with someone about a stressful or troublesome event in your life. This conversation releases the burdens from situations that crowd your mind. Letting go of your drama will allow you to breathe normally again and feel a sense of freedom from fear and hurt. It also allows you to get valuable feedback from the person you confide in.

If you don't have a friend or family member you wish to confide in, then consider church groups, peer groups, and even a therapist.

For all you cold-climate dwellers, here's an analogy for you: Think about when you come indoors to a heated room from the outside freezing cold temperature. You're wearing layers of clothing causing you to be hot and extremely uncomfortable. Upon entering your warm home, you quickly rip off the layers of clothing that confine you so that your body can adjust to the new temperature. Isn't this the best feeling? By tearing off the layers, you create a new body temperature and freedom of movement that is so much more comfortable for you. You can't do this with your coat on, just like you can't lose weight when you have layers of negative thoughts in your head or negative energy in your body. When you confide in someone you trust, you get to rip off the emotional layers that impede your progress. Uncluttering your mind allows your body to achieve more physical comfort and your mind more space to commit to your weight loss journey. Are you ready to take off your layers? Then speak your mind.

EXERCISES

(1) Who is my confidant?

(2) Have I considered looking into therapy before?

(3) Does my health insurance cover a therapist?

TOOL 21. ADDRESS EXTERNAL ADVERSITY

I know it's overwhelming when you lack the right support system from the key people in your life. This is the hardest thing to come to terms with, but if your spouse, family member, coworker, or best friend doesn't support your weight-loss journey, then you must address this. Be okay with the fact that it's not their responsibility to help you lose weight. It's yours. You owe it to yourself to be real about what you want. But you're the one who must do the work.

Don't allow anyone to affect your weight-loss plan. If you've had a weight-loss saboteur your entire life, then figure out a viable way to succeed at losing weight while addressing the adversity this person causes you.

I worked with a woman whose husband would always bring sweets into the house, and she always ended up eating most of the food. She lacked self-control. He insisted on having this food in the house and told her that he shouldn't have to be victim to her diet. He told her to learn self-control. She ended up asking him why he was so adverse to her weight-loss goal. She heard him out. After putting her defensive barrier down, she realized that her husband felt abandoned by her new lifestyle plan. He is overweight himself. He felt that his wife wouldn't spend quality time with him anymore over a glass of wine with cheese, crackers, and chocolate. So, now what?

In this case, she could assure her spouse that she would bond over wine and cheese once a week. She decided that this weekly plan would be her free meal and her time to bond with her hubby. It's a win-win. Even though she's technically "cheating" four times a month instead of the two free days I suggested earlier, it's still a solid plan of action that works for her today.

Again, this is your journey and your plan. Other options in a similar situation might be motivating your spouse to eat healthier by cooking scrumptious, enjoyable meals. You could also sign up together for a healthy gourmet cooking class, take evening walks with him or her, or give your spouse a five-minute shoulder massage and debrief each night. The goal is to go to bed with a restful mind. You are working toward establishing a healthier way of life with the person you love, too.

For some people, adopting a healthy lifestyle breaks a special bond with someone. I understand that this is a huge challenge. You must pursue good health while preserving your relationships with these people through alternative outlets. If friends and family still make this challenging for you, then perhaps seeing them on specific days of the week will keep you on track. One cheat meal with a friend or family member every couple of weeks won't throw you off, remember? Afterward, you'll go right back on track the very next meal.

Don't resent the people you love for their lack of support. Sometimes people are envious or even lack the tools to be supportive. Sometimes they fear change and don't want to be a part of your change. I recently told a patient to clear out his pantry of all the cookies and crackers. He told me that he's keeping these things around for his grandchildren. I told him that he must lead by example and teach his grandchildren healthier behaviors. He hesitated and told me he'll think about it. I informed him that childhood obesity has become a rampant epidemic. Parents and grandparents can help experts like me lower the incidences of childhood obesity by instilling healthy practices in their homes.

No one but you can make these changes for you. Live to be the best you for you. Without hurting anyone or feeling resentful toward anyone, choose a healthier way of life for yourself.

EXERCISES

(1) Who causes me external adversity? How?

(2) What are my top three goals for my conversation with them?

(3) What are some potential responses from them that I must prepare for?

(4) How can I engage in a successful conversation without upsetting anyone?

TOOL 22. SCHEDULE DAILY "ME" TIME

Let's decide that, moving forward, you'll never let a day go by without giving yourself at least thirty minutes of *me* time. At the end of every day, you go home with yourself, live in your body and own your own thoughts. You must, therefore, put yourself first because no one else will. No matter what job you have, how many kids you have, or how demanding your partner is, scheduling *me* time is very important. This means no phone calls, no external conversations, and no distractions. Just you, somewhere out there for thirty minutes or more a day.

As someone who loves working out, my *me* time is sometimes spent at the gym. For example, I was swamped with work one day, and I still went to the gym. I spent thirty minutes lifting weights. When I was going there, I remember thinking, "This is out of the way and I have so much to do." However, I was able to get my full workout in and as always I felt amazing afterward. You must put being healthy high on your priority list.

Having daily *me* time gives you a feeling of importance in this world. You may choose to exercise in your *me* time. Exercise keeps your body young by circulating the blood and keeping hormone secretion higher. You can spend these thirty minutes in a different way every day. One day you can go watch the sunset and meditate (two tools in one—yeah, baby!) You can take a new class at the gym, go to the farmer's market, or shop for a size down. Spend your time wisely. What you do in this time must make sense for your weight-loss journey.

EXERCISES

(1) What did I do for myself today during *me* time?

(2) How did this help me progress toward my weight-loss goal?

(3) Which other three tools will I use to accommodate my *me* time this week?

TOOL 23. GET RID OF JEALOUSY

The competition stops right now. You are out of the competition with others and now get to be with yourself. Don't be against yourself; be *with* yourself. If you don't compare yourself to others, you're ahead. Otherwise, pay close attention. Jealousy is a sign of insecurity. There's a reason for this. When you're off-balance and not happy with yourself, you tend to look at what others have and envy them. Envy can be hostile and actually a waste of your energy. Envy clutters your mind with negative thoughts about life, which will only be fed by a poor body image, negative energy, and overeating.

I'm not saying that all people who experience jealousy are out causing confrontations, but jealous people have a recognizable communication style that is very dark toward others. People can feel your energy, so don't fool yourself. Jealousy isolates people both emotionally and physically. When you're in isolation, you feed the monster whatever it wants.

You will often turn to food to feel fulfilled. Envy can lead to other addictions such as drinking, drugs, and gambling.

Envy will only make you weaker, never stronger. It is a character trait that must be resolved if you really want to succeed in any journey. Getting rid of it actually makes you more fun to be around, too. Figure out why you're jealous of whomever. Is it because he's more successful? Is it because she drives a nicer car than you do? Is it because his children go to private school? Getting ahead in life requires hard work. Hard workers possess perseverance. I don't often meet successful people who are envious. If you work hard for everything you want, then eventually you may get it. The question is, are you willing to follow through until you get it? Hard workers will.

Ditch the jealousy and start enhancing your own life. Realize that everyone possesses different levels of financial security, resources, and opportunities. Some of us were raised to work hard for everything we've got, and others were given everything they have. Either way, who cares? Why waste your energy being jealous of someone else when you could put all your energy into bettering yourself? If you want something and don't have it, then work for it. You wanna be lean? Then do the work.

My friend Meg, whom I love so dearly, had the picture-perfect life when I first met her eight years ago. She already owned a condo and made good money. As we grew closer, I realized people were very envious of what she had. What people don't realize is how hard this girl works and how grueling her responsibilities are each day. People see a gorgeous girl who owns a home in the hills, has an amazing child, is happily married, and possesses a lot of beautiful things in her life. Meg works her butt off for it all. To this day, I feel so proud of her. She is now one of my best friends, and we both work at inspiring each other. She and I meet every December to reflect on the past year's goals as we set the New Year's goals for the year ahead.

Be inspired and befriend great people in your life. Offer them a synergistic relationship the way Meg and I do for each other. If jealousy finds you again, check it at the door. Shift your energy away from jealousy and work harder for your goals in life. Life is full of potential. Focus on what you have versus what you don't have. Focus on exhausting your potential instead of exhausting your mind with envy.

Take a moment to reflect on your top five gifts that life has given you so far. You may then write a different list of the top five gifts you wish you had. Write out a plan so that you can ultimately work the plan. Find someone you love to be your sounding board.

EXERCISES

(1) What five gifts do I have?

(2) What five gifts do I want?

(3) Who am I jealous of and why?

(4) How will I dump this jealousy?

TOOL 24. LEARN HUMILITY

Humility is defined as the condition of being humble. When you have unrealistic expectations of yourself each day, you're fighting humility. You may overload your mind with clutter, making life seem unbearable. Learn how to be humble so that you can deal with life's surprises with minimal stress.

Don't be vulnerable to the world's judgments of you. Don't take things too seriously. As my client Bud once told me, "Don't sweat the small stuff." By that, he meant everything is small. You never need to accept unsolicited advice from anyone.

Learn how to channel your thoughts into your own trials and tribulations. I find that people offer insight into other people's issues rather than handling their own. Learn *what* is holding you back from change and *how* to change it. Learn to accept where you are today, and plan on where you want to go tomorrow. Be accountable. This is humility.

Ask yourself why you haven't lost your weight yet. Identify *how* you can lose your weight. Write your answers down. This place of self-realization is up to you. No weight-loss fairy will arrive at your doorstep with these answers. It's within you. Trust yourself. Dig inside of yourself to figure it out. Maybe you can relate to one of the scenarios below.

SCENARIO 1

You've tried losing twenty-five pounds for more than six months now. You lost the first ten pounds and then you started traveling, which threw you off plan.

BASIC FACTS

What: Traveling spoils your weight-loss journey.

How: Long hours on the road spoil your eating habits and you're too tired to exercise.

Solution: Bring protein shake packets, protein bars, and a healthy sandwich on whole-grain toast (you have my permission to eat bread when traveling on a plane) with three ounces of lean-cut meat, lots of vegetables, and no dressing. Bring a piece of fruit and some almonds. When you land, look for a small convenience store so that you can purchase water and some healthy groceries for your room. Make the decision to find good nutrition wherever you go. Find the hotel gym. If there's no gym, then go for a walk. Walk the hotel stairs by staying on a higher floor.

SCENARIO 2

You joined a diet center and got sick halfway through the program. When the program ended, the diet center said that you had to buy more time to continue with the program. You decided to quit because you'd put all your weight back on and don't want to spend more money to get it off again.

BASIC FACTS

What: You got sick and didn't get to finish the plan.

How: The time expired and you have to buy more treatment.

Solution: Ask the center if you can bring in a doctor's note so that you can pick up where you left off. If they don't agree to this, then make a deal with them to purchase the difference between the remaining weeks that were unused in your program from the time you used it before getting sick. This is worth it if it means successfully losing and keeping the weight off. You can also consider asking for a partial refund. There are always options in these types of situations. Pick an option and then stick to it. Express your true desire to be there. Show some humility. But whatever you do, don't you dare quit!

SCENARIO 3

You've been eating healthy, but your loved one is still eating poorly and drinking booze. He or she has expressed loneliness to you since your new lifestyle is different from the one he or she is used to. Even though you're willing to teach your loved one the fundamentals of healthy eating, this person continues to buy fattening things, like your favorite ice cream. You find yourself falling off because it's hard to resist.

BASIC FACTS

What: Two different lifestyles under one roof.

How: Your significant other continues to be unhealthy.

Solution: There are many things to do here. Let's look at three options.

(1) Get your significant other to be healthy with you.

(2) Introduce modified/healthier versions of what he or she loves to eat. For example, instead of a tuna salad sandwich, try a tuna salad lettuce wrap with

pepperoncinis(spicy peppers), cucumbers, tomatoes, and half an avocado instead of mayonnaise. Yummy!

(3) Get another refrigerator and put it in the garage for his or her "stuff" so that you never need to look at it. Only healthy food belongs in the kitchen, right?

EXERCISES

(1) What is my first step to attaining humility?

(2) What is holding me back from achieving it?

(3) Why haven't I achieved my goal weight yet?

(4) What is a sample scenario that I face? What are the **what, how,** and **solution** similar to the examples above?

TOOL 25. LEARN TO SAY NO

No one wants to hear the word *no*, which is why most people don't even say it. It symbolizes denial and rejection. *No* is like a huge stop sign in front of your face that sends you to a screeching halt. *No* is that annoying hand held in front of your face while you're conversing with someone who's reactive in their communication style. The word *no* can promote confrontation. If *no* is this powerful, then why don't people use it against saboteurs? From now on, when someone offers you candy at work, say no thanks. When your family offers you unhealthy food, just say no thanks. When you're at a restaurant and they ask you if you want bread or dessert, say no thanks. You get my drift?

Let's take this a step further. Learn to say no to the tasks that aren't high priority for you. Learn to unclutter your mind and simplify your days with things that fit into *your* schedule. Don't overload your schedule with the things others want you to do for them.

Let's take one of my clients, for example. She never says no to friends. As a result, she is very overwhelmed and overweight. One day, she got pulled away from her own household responsibilities to help a friend clean her garage. This forced her to give up her own responsibilities, which left her with no other window of time to get her own chores done that week. She should have told her friend, "I cannot help you today, but how about next Monday?" In this kind of a situation, pick a day that works for you. Otherwise, you're duping yourself.

It's all in your presentation of the word *no*. Don't be rude. Be honest. For example, in the above scenario, you could say to your friend, "I really hate chores like cleaning out the garage, and I'm not great at organizing. Could we do something else together?" Put yourself first moving forward, and don't feel guilty. Your intentions aren't to ever hurt anyone. Establish your own limits in life. The goal is to feel like there's room for more. Always keep your proverbial plate only three-quarters full. The remaining room is for fitness and good health. Learn to step back. Learning to say no means taking control of your life and creating room for personal growth.

EXERCISES

(1) What is one thing this week that I should have said *no* to?

(2) Why do I fear the word *no*?

(3) Since using this tool, what healthy habit(s) have I added?

TOOL 26. MARCH TO YOUR OWN BEAT

We get to travel the road of life for a short period of time. This is why we must each learn to march to the beat of our own drum. When you move very fast all the time, it's like sprinting really fast despite the fact that your body is running out of "juice." A lifestyle spent in the fast lane wears you down to the bone. Think more about running a marathon: steady, precise, and longer in duration. I'm not suggesting that you lose momentum, but learn how to develop the stamina and mental agility to transition over to a more manageable beat. Many people lead lives that are similar to the Energizer bunny. Unfortunately, that isn't a realistic rhythm.

Your lifestyle choices are causing you to be overweight. Your body was not built to handle the stressors of modern-day society. The fitness industry has developed a million and one messages for you to learn from. Are your eyes, ears, and mind open to these messages? Start looking into why your mind is racing. Why race? Life's finish line won't reward you with a medal—just a tombstone.

Make your life purposeful. Change what you can, and modify your perception of the things you can't. Learn the lifestyle of a healthy person and choose to live this way. Once you acquire a lean body, you'll see how rewarding it is to be lean, and you'll want to maintain this forever. Start today by discovering the power behind living in a fit body, and you'll enter the gateways of a whole new world. There's no need to feel powerless as you evolve. Powerless energy leads to overconsumption of food, lack of activity, and negative thoughts. Nothing will get done under these circumstances. Every day should involve positive thoughts about your journey.

Great example: I have a highly social client who lost twenty-three pounds within six months. In the second six months, he only lost five pounds. Most people would be discouraged by this. However, in marching to the beat of his own drum, he is still the master of his lifestyle and will proceed with his weight-loss journey over the course of time. To date, he has lost a total of thirty-six pounds. He is only nine pounds away from reaching his goal. He took fourteen months to get to this point. Even though this seems long, he is what I call a successful loser.

It's okay to lose weight slowly. I prefer it, actually. You will lose from the right places when you lose slowly. Losing slowly is healthier, too. Be real with yourself and modify your lifestyle where needed. Find your own beat. Your rhythm is yours. Own it.

EXERCISES

(1) What is my rhythm for this week?

(2) If I could change anything about the pace of my day, what would I change?

(3) How will I change this aspect of my day?

TOOL 27. TAKE A PERSONAL DAY

In addition to scheduling *me* time for yourself every day (tool 22), take at least one day off every quarter. Don't pride yourself on not taking any vacation or sick time because companies don't reward you for this. Your health should be the most valuable asset to you. Tell your company in advance so that it makes business sense. Just be responsible.

Personal days refuel your mind so that you're more productive at work the next day. This day belongs to you. I find that most people who struggle with weight loss are the ones who fail to give themselves a day to unwind and reflect on what their own needs are.

Losing weight requires a healthy outlook on life and lots of rest, relaxation, and self-love. If you're constantly under the gun at work and your personal life is one big rollercoaster ride, then it's time to learn new strategies and tools to help redirect your lifestyle. You must change the things that no

74

longer work for you. Only you can determine what those things are. Remember, your weight symbolizes your lifestyle and reflects your level of self-respect. Recognize that it takes the mindset of strength to rebuild a healthier you. The mindset is set by your own thoughts and the type of thoughts you wish to engage in each day. One way of strengthening your mindset to a more positive outlook is to take a personal day for mental and emotional reflection.

Don't schedule anything else that will occupy your time on this day. Start the day off by catching up with yourself. Set your intentions for the week ahead. Sit down with your goal sheet and ask yourself what tools you need today to better yourself for tomorrow. Set up time frames to get things done (tool 75). Determine how you will measure your success.

Personal days are all about you. Don't give them up to someone else. Here are some ideas for what a personal day can look like:

- Treat yourself to the spa.

- Go shopping.

- Start your goal sheet.

- Go to the beach.

- Take a road trip.

- Stay home and do nothing at all.

- Clean your home.

- Work out.

- Participate in a workshop.

- Go hiking and have a picnic at the top of the mountain.

- Schedule your doctor appointments and get on top of your health.

- Schedule something from your bucket list (tool 101).

- Drive to a nice place.

You might even choose to be spontaneous about what you do. That's okay. Treat this day like a gift. This day will give you room for self-discovery. It will allow you to measure how your annual goals are progressing. Remember, successful weight loss is a lifelong commitment. Successful weight loss might mean giving up some of the things you enjoy—but only those things that are keeping you overweight.

EXERCISES

(1) When are my scheduled personal days?

(2) Of the 107 tools presented in this book, how many did I use for my personal day?

(3) Which tools have I truly mastered overall?

TOOL 28. KEEP A DAILY FOOD JOURNAL

Virtually every person I know who keeps a food journal succeeds at weight loss. I know you've heard this advice before. It isn't new. But we don't do it often enough. Let me reiterate what other fitness and health-care experts have been trying to tell you all along: Keeping a daily journal will help you lose weight. It will hold you accountable for truthful meal intake and map out what's going on each day—the type of exercise you did, how much fluid you consumed, and how much sleep you got each night. It will also track your frequency of small meal consumption (tool 31) throughout the day. I'm a big believer that four to five small meals a day eventually burns the fat away. Journaling also allows you to identify which food combinations and portions achieve balance for you.

Most people don't like keeping a journal. I say that's due to laziness. Don't be lazy. A daily journal is your time to reflect on your achievements for the day. You can even personalize your journal by adding in daily quotes and positive affirmations. A daily journal allows you to be conscious of your own behaviors. The more conscious you are, the more likely you'll be able to form good habits.

I've learned that people may think they're eating right, but their portions are way too large. It's time to be real with yourself. There's something called the Hawthorne effect when people tend to behave because they know they're being watched. Keeping a journal forces you to record the truth, unless you consciously decide to negate some of the truth. But then again, who are you fooling, right? If you decide to eat a piece of cake one day, then you might as well log it. This journal should identify the catalysts that drive you to behave the way you do. It will help you identify if you're eating the right amounts of each macronutrient (fats, proteins, and carbohydrates) or if you're overeating. You will be able to identify the highs and lows in your energy, any improvement in daily activities, any weight loss, and which food combinations satiate you most.

Wonderful Web sites are available to help you count calories and macronutrients. Your cell phone may also have a weight-loss application for you to use. Do a Google search for "free food journals" and review your options. You can even write your journal down in a notebook.

Regardless of your method, the number-one secret is consistency. Inconsistency will not result in good weight loss. Consistency means being great for months at a time until your healthy behaviors become habit. A lot of people I've coached in the past will be on one week and off one week, on for one month and off for two weeks. This is not consistency. Consistency is following through with healthy behaviors every day and allowing for two free days a month (tool 18) if needed.

Log your food, fitness, and lifestyle behaviors for at least four consecutive weeks. Do not miss a day. Be real with your log. Remember, this journal is for you so that you can succeed at losing weight.

Below is an unmodified, detailed journal from one of my male clients who has attained his goal. Please note that his goals were primarily fat loss, and that all of his supplements were prescribed by a physician. He had lab tests run to determine which supplements to take. I'm impressed with his attention to detail in his journal, which is why I'm sharing it with you. He felt honored that I asked him to put his journal in my book. I call him the lean mean fighting machine. His journal was logged throughout the day on his blackberry so he didn't have to log it all at night. His attention to detail was his way of staying in tuned with his needs. You will note that he not only logs his nutrition but also includes a daily intention, quote, his sleep patterns, and his exercise regiment for the day. He is very in touch with his entire lifestyle including how his body feels, which is why he attained his goal and continues to do well. Not everyone keeps as detailed of a journal. As long as you log your portions, indicate what you ate, what time you ate, what type of exercise you accomplished, how much water you drank, how much sleep you got and reflect on having *me* time every day, you are good to go.

> **This Week's Intention/Goals:** *1) This week is a week to calm down and focus on my goals. 2) To calm the mind in the face of significant change is a necessary skill needed to take it to the next level. 3) There will be big changes in 2012 and I must be mentally prepared.*
>
> **Today's Quote:** *"Life isn't about finding yourself. Life is about creating yourself." (George Bernard Shaw)*
>
> **Sleep:** *8:45 p.m.–3:45 a.m. (solid): 7 hrs.*
>
> **Weight (upon rising):** *177.6 lbs. (trend: steady)*
>
> **Injuries/Soreness:** *all good*
>
> *04:00 a.m.: 8 oz. fresh Colombian black coffee plain; 4 oz. water*
>
> *06:00 a.m.: MEAL #1: (6 eggs) 2 eggs whole, 4 egg whites—plain, ½ avocado, small handful of sunflower seeds; 2 fish oil tabs; 20 oz. water*
>
> *06:30 a.m.: Morning Supplements: (1) antioxidant supplements (2) multivitamin packet; (3) vitamin D3 5,000 IU; 12 oz. water*

07:00 a.m.: 32 oz. water

08:30 a.m.: Protein shake

10:00 a.m.: MEAL #2: 2/3 cup organic lentils, 2/3 cup ground sirloin (crumbled), small handful of walnut pieces, handful of baby spinach, 1/2 avocado; 2 fish oil tabs; 28 oz. water

12:00 pm: 8 oz. oolong tea; handful of raw almonds

02:00 p.m.: MEAL #3: 4 oz. skinless chicken breast, 1 cup of raw broccoli, 1 teaspoon of all-natural peanut butter; 2 fish oil tabs; 20 oz. water

04:00 p.m.: MEAL #4: 4 egg whites, 1/2 cup organic butter beans, 2 tablespoons ground sirloin, 2 cups of spinach salad with light oil-and-vinegar dressing; 1 teaspoon peanut butter for dessert; 12 oz. water

05:00 p.m.: Protein shake

07:00 p.m.: Evening supplement regimen: (1) Magnesium Orotate, 500 mg; (2) Progesterone; (3) Melatonin, 2 mg; (4) DHEA, 50 mg; (5) 8 oz. water

Below is a much simpler food journal from another client. Even though this journal is less detailed than the previous one, this client still got fabulous results. He lost fifteen pounds of fat and gained ten pounds of muscle in three months. The food journal helped me coach him every single day which is why his results are awesome.

Log

5:00 a.m.

30 minutes on the elliptical trainer. Performed interval program at level 10

6:00 a.m.

Protein shake-(30 grams) with one cup of mixed berries

8:00 a.m.

Cottage cheese with one full cucumber, and 1/2 hand full sunflower seeds

10:00 a.m.

Tangerine and 1/2 handful of almonds

12:30 p.m.

20 oz. green drink: kale, spinach, celery, parsley, cucumber, green apple, and ginger

1:30 p.m.

4 oz. salmon, a scoop of egg salad, and one whole cucumber

3:30 p.m.

1/2 pear, Greek yogurt, 1/2 cup of berries

5:00 p.m.

1/2 cup cottage cheese with dried apricot

7:00 p.m.

Breast of chicken with cauliflower, broccoli, one small sweet potato, green beans, and mixed green salad

9:00 p.m.

Pear 1/2 handful of almonds

Keeping a food journal allows you to reflect on your day at the end of your day. This helps you track your intake while feeling proud of your healthy accomplishments for the day.

EXERCISES

(1) Does my cell phone have a food log application?

(2) How will I log my food? (Stick to one method.)

(3) What have I learned from journaling?

(4) Who will I show my log to?

TOOL 29. IMPROVE YOUR SLEEP

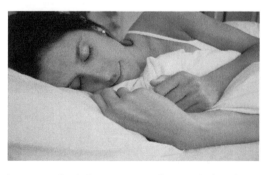

Without a good night's rest, your body won't function normally and it will suffer the next day. Sleep deprivation contributes to obesity. Your body requires sleep to repair itself. Sleep is also needed for a sound mind, body, and soul. When you don't get adequate sleep each night, you fail to repair your cells from oxidative stress, and you can't kill off bacteria or viruses in your body. Sleep deprivation also exacerbates your cravings for sugar and salt the next day.

Symptoms of poor sleep include the following:

- Irritability

- Constipation

- Increased cravings

- Low concentration and mental acuity

- Low motivation

- Depression

- Anxiety

- Very low energy

- Decreased weight loss

- Increased cellular damage

It's recommended that you sleep at least seven hours a night. Everyone is different though. Unfortunately, nothing has been confirmed. I can safely suggest that the more you challenge your body through mental, physical, or emotional work, the longer you'll need to recharge your battery at night.

Time isn't the only factor to consider. Quality of sleep is key. It's imperative to accomplish deep REM sleep when you sleep. Getting up in the middle of the night disturbs the quality of sleep. Therefore, avoid fluids two hours before bedtime; otherwise, you'll be up several times a night to use the bathroom. If you're thirsty at night, simply wet your lips without drinking a whole glass of fluid.

Sleep deprivation is a concern for not only adults but children, too. High sugar consumption or high-glycemic carbs before bedtime will hinder sleep. In general, high-sugar nutrition contributes to hormonal and physiological imbalances. High sugar instigates explosive levels of insulin in the bloodstream, which I mention all throughout this book. This will devastate your weight-loss results. When you sleep poorly, you subconsciously reach for lots of sugar all throughout the next day just to boost your energy levels. It's ultimately up to you to reestablish the right internal physiology so that you can sleep better. Be patient with this process because you're undoing years of poor habits that take time to change.

Your activities before bedtime may also be to blame. Keep your mind under-stimulated prior to bedtime. Consider avoiding the following activities before bedtime:

- Heavy computer usage

- Watching television (Blue light can disturb your ability to sleep.)

- Caffeinated beverages after noon

- Alcohol consumption

- An argument or other emotional discussion

- Heavy exercise

- Business planning

Sometimes, no matter how hard we try, our minds run a race right before we go to sleep. Keep a pad and pen out by your bed and defer your thoughts onto paper for the next day. This can help you transition into a restful state.

There is also a physical cause for lack of sleep. During sleep apnea, a sleeping disorder, there are pauses in breathing patterns while you sleep. These pauses can occur many times an hour and deprive your brain of oxygen. You may not be aware of your own sleep apnea, but other people such as a spouse can hear it. If there's any question regarding whether or not you have sleep apnea, ask your doctor. Sleep apnea is a serious medical disorder that needs immediate medical attention. It can put you at risk for cardiovascular disease, headaches, memory loss, and depression. People with sleep apnea feel very tired every day and may not even know why. This disorder can cause you to eat more during the day, which will impede weight loss. Don't take this lightly.

Remember, poor sleep always results in poor weight loss. If you have truly applied all of the above recommendations prior to bedtime and still have trouble sleeping, then talk to your doctor until you find the right answer. Help yourself sleep peacefully through the night.

EXERCISES

(1) Which activities should I cut out before bedtime?

(2) On a scale of 1 to 10, 1 being poor and 10 being great, how would I rate my energy levels when I wake up?

TOOL 30. TAKE PHOTOS OF EACH MEAL

Have you ever kept a written food journal (tool 28) for a fitness or nutrition coach and felt that it was a waste of time because you weren't losing weight? Well, no offense, but many times food journals are completely inaccurate. Most dieters don't report what they're actually eating because they're scared of getting in trouble with their "coach." Hiring a coach shouldn't feel like the good old days when you went to the principal's office. You're not in trouble. Don't be afraid to admit if you made a mistake. If you fall off, simply get right back on. No need to hide the truth.

Be honest with yourself. When you keep a food journal, you lose weight. If you're not losing weight quickly enough, don't get discouraged. People lose at different rates—be patient. If you're simply overeating and don't realize it, taking pictures of your food can help your coach help you. For example, I worked with a client who said she was eating oatmeal and peanut butter for breakfast every morning. That sounds okay until you see the ice cream scoop of peanut butter she was plopping onto her oatmeal. This is not acceptable for someone who wants to lose weight. While two tablespoons of peanut butter equates to 14 grams of fat and 180 calories, her portion looked like it was at least triple that. Can you imagine consuming 42 grams of fat and 540 calories of peanut butter alone, not including the oatmeal? That'll never be the formula for weight loss, I promise you.

I started requesting picture journals from clients who aren't succeeding. I get to "see" exactly what their meal looks like. Most people think they know what healthy eating is, but many don't. Don't ignore this if this is you. Learning is easier than you think. For example, do you ever eat cereal and fat-free milk for breakfast? Well, low and behold, most cereals possess more than 40 grams of high-glycemic carbohydrates, which causes your blood sugar to spike. The sugar in your cereal doesn't even include the sugar from the milk. Also, most cereals are only three-quarters of a cup per serving. Stop for a moment. Go into your cabinet and pull out the measuring cup. Grab your cereal and pour it into the cup. That's what I said: "That's it?" Portion control is vital; otherwise you'll consume too many carbohydrates, mainly from refined carbohydrates, which will spike your blood sugars. This will keep you fat.

Another client of mine said that he ate *very* well and completely understood how to eat healthy. Pictures showed me that he was consuming a twelve-ounce steak, a small potato, and three stalks of asparagus (if his wife remembered to serve him the vegetable) for dinner. To most Americans, this is a perfect dinner. However, your body won't absorb all that protein, only a third, if that. Very rarely do we see a four-ounce steak available. No one ever needs a twelve-ounce steak—unless you're one of my boys from Gold's Gym in Venice Beach.

Make sure you eat lots of veggies and stay away from high-glycemic carbohydrates (tool 68) after six p.m. as a general rule of thumb (you can do a sweet potato or yam). Even if you didn't eat your small meals throughout the day, that doesn't mean that you should eat high-calorie meals at night. Dinner should be your lowest-calorie meal so that your body isn't stuffed before bedtime. Sleep is when your engine gets turned off completely.

Eat small, frequent meals throughout the day. Taking pictures of your food will help keep your portions right and your awareness high for adopting new, healthy eating habits.

EXERCISES

(1) Do I have a camera or cell phone that takes clear pictures?

_____

(2) Who can check my picture food log for me?

_____

Chapter 3

YOUR BODY IS YOUR TEMPLE

The mind and the body operate like best friends. If one is off, the other is affected. These systems want to get along, but their synergy relies heavily on your everyday behaviors. It's up to you to treat your body like a temple. If you neglect your body, then your mind will be negatively affected. This isn't a good formula for good health. It's definitely not good for weight loss. The following tools will help you produce a powerful body that is topped by a sound mind.

TOOL 31. EAT SMALL FREQUENT MEALS

Most people skip breakfast, run to work, and are awake for hours before consuming their first meal. Other people eat a very large breakfast, skip lunch and binge at dinner. Both scenarios will result in weight issues. The body is not built to be flooded with calories at any particular meal, let alone at night. When you skip meals throughout the day and eat very large meals, not only will your body store what it doesn't use, but it will also hold onto fat all day long. I know, not cool!

It's time to respect the way your body operates. When you wake up in the morning, your body's metabolic engine starts up and is ready to drive. Do you want to drive without gas in your engine? Heck no! Where do you think your body is getting the fuel from if you're not eating breakfast? Certainly not from fat. In addition, you reduce your RMR (tool 49) as a result of long periods in between meals. Putting your body into mini-starvation cycles during the day never works. Small frequent meals feed your mind and body throughout the day providing you with better energy, better mental acuity, greater moods, and successful weight loss. Isn't this what you want? When you consume the correct portions and satiate your body throughout the day, you lose weight. Your body eventually acclimates to this schedule and provides you with the signals to eat again, which is anywhere between three to four hours later. Once the sun begins to set, your body is ready to settle into its natural circadian rhythm, ready for sleep. When you don't eat small frequent meals throughout the day, you'll over-eat at night, which disturbs your sleep and weight loss success.

So, what if you're not hungry four to five times a day? What if you're not hungry when you wake up? First, ban the what if attitude and welcome the change (tool 13). This is all part of the process of breaking the chains of obesity. The word breakfast sounds like breaking a fast, right? Keep a food journal (tool 28) and realize that your body needs small frequent meals throughout the day to avoid overeating.

What should each meal look like? Everyone is different but the basics apply. Remember to visit tool 59 to see how much protein you should consume. The rest of your meals should consist of healthy fats (tool 56), vegetables and fruits (tool 60). Allow yourself to break your chains through low glycemic nutrition (tool 68) which has never failed when followed closely. Consider hiring a coach to guide you through this change. You are worth the investment.

Here is a sample healthy day:

Breakfast: one protein, a fruit, and vegetables. One grain if you train in the a.m.

e.g.: Egg-white omelet with onions, peppers, broccoli, zucchini, and sliced tomatoes; 1 cup of berries. Optional ½ cup of oatmeal.

Snack: one protein and a vegetable (Fruit is optional.)
e.g.: One scoop of protein powder blended with one kale bunch, one cucumber, parsley, ginger, and an apple.

Lunch: one protein, vegetables, and a healthy fat.
e.g.: Two cups of spinach, one heirloom tomato, one cucumber, two teaspoons of walnuts, half an avocado, and organic chicken breast.

Snack: one protein, fruit, and optional healthy fat.
e.g.: Low-fat cottage cheese with 1/2 cup of berries with ten almonds.

Dinner: one protein and veggies galore.
e.g.: Chilean sea bass with fresh lemon served with one cup of steamed asparagus, and one sweet potato (which is actually considered a low glycemic carb.) With this, have a huge green dinner salad with two tablespoons of dressing.

EXERCISES

(1) How many meals do I currently eat a day?

(2) What is my biggest barrier to eating small frequent meals?

(3) What is my plan of action to eliminate this barrier?

TOOL 32. SCHEDULE EXERCISE

A to-do list will unclutter your head (tool 1). I'm very old-school. I never relied on a Palm Pilot (remember those?) or any other electronic toy to track my life in. I like the feeling of writing down my daily goals and physically putting a check mark next to each item when I finish a task. I own an "At-a-Glance" daily planner that holds all of my daily lists for my career, training sessions, Spin classes, boot camp classes, educational courses, lectures, and other appointments. I log scheduled phone calls, anecdotal notes, thoughts, the names of people I spoke with, people's birthdays, and other reminders. This works for me. If you prefer a different logging tool, then go right ahead and use it.

Schedule your exercise appointments in your weekly planner, too. I know you probably have the intention of exercising. Committing to specific times and days in your planner will actually make it happen. Lack of planning sets you up for inactivity. Determine a realistic amount of times you'll exercise each week. Schedule it and then show up for it. That's it.

People say they lack time. I believe that people lack the motivation to make time. If you have no time for good health, then good luck finding time later when you have no choice but to see your doctor for a sedentary-induced disease. Your body is your vehicle for getting around, remember? Exercise lubes your joints and keeps your engine running optimally.

One of my clients is a nurse for the Red Cross and works a lot of overtime hours, so she was having trouble finding time to go to the gym. After probing, I found out that she has three days a week to commit to the gym. She always gets into work at ten a.m. on Wednesdays and Thursdays. She doesn't work on

Saturdays. With this schedule, I instructed her to make those three days her workout days. Voila! We have a plan for her.

Life needs to contain movement. We were hunters and gatherers. We only sat down after a full day of running around catching our own food. Now, half of the country sits for more than half of their day and food is delivered to them. Sitting is one of the worst postures you can be in all day long. Sitting causes lower back pain because your lower back and legs get tight. We are bipedal animals. Your legs were designed to generate blood flow back to the heart by walking and running. Sitting handicaps the legs from moving blood back to your heart. Your arteries will eventually stiffen and become diseased. You can prevent this through moving more each day and exercising each week.

Schedule your week so that you have a plan. Here are some *sample* exercise plans:

Vigorous week: Three days of one-hour interval training and four days of strength training. Add yoga and/or a martial art into this mix. Stretch on non-yoga days. This program is for the person who isn't new to exercise.

Less-vigorous week: Two days of circuit training, one day of yoga, and two days of 45-minute cardio-group classes such as Spinning®, indoor rowing, or kickboxing. Stretch on non-yoga days. This is for the person who trains inconsistently but has been doing something and wants to deepen their commitment.

Even-less-vigorous week: Three days of circuit training (e.g.: M-W-F or Tu-Th-Sat) with a twenty-minute high incline treadmill walk to finish. Stretch. This is for the person who hasn't been exercising for three months or more.

Beginner week: Walk thirty minutes a day five days a week. Stretch. This is for the person who is just starting and should add weight training in 2-4 weeks.

These are sample workout schedules to choose from. You will notice that each week differs for you, so set a realistic schedule for yourself at the beginning of each week and then stick to it. Definitely wear a heart-rate monitor when you train. If you're a beginner, then use a pedometer. If you haven't tested your VO_2 max yet (tool 42), consider using this formula: *220 – age – resting heart rate x 65–85 percent effort of your max heart rate + resting heart rate = your active heart rate*. For the percent effort of your max heart rate, multiply only one value at a time, whether it's 65 percent or higher. Take your resting heart rate when you first wake up in the morning. Using your pointer and middle fingers, find your pulse on the thumb side of your wrist or carotid artery in your neck. Count the beats for one full minute. That is your resting heart rate.

It's time to exercise consistently! No more excuses. Just make it happen!

EXERCISES

(1) Which days and times will I exercise this week?

(2) What exercise regimen do I feel comfortable doing?

(3) Where will I exercise?

TOOL 33. CREATE AN ACCOUNTABILITY SYSTEM

Taking tool 32 a step further, once you schedule your exercise for the week, you must follow through with the plan. For every time you follow through with exercise, you could reward yourself with something pleasurable that week. Practice the concept of positive reinforcement for a strong accountability system for yourself. If you're in the habit of rewarding yourself already without a reason, then that's where you'll need to shift. For example, ladies, from now on, every week you participate in exercise and good nutrition, treat yourself to a spa pedicure, massage, new pair of shoes, or anything that brings you enjoyment. Men, every time you exercise, treat yourself to a golf game or something that brings you excitement. You should only reward yourself when you exercise and partake in healthy lifestyle habits.

It's up to you to follow through with this tool. The internet makes it easy to access virtually anything you want. Think back to your childhood days when you had to complete a task or finish a chore before earning a sticker or new toy. That's accountability. You must relearn how to remain disciplined throughout this journey. It's time to relearn the positive reinforcement system by only rewarding your healthy behaviors, moving forward.

I don't want this book to be just another fluffy read in which you ignore the strategies for change. Therefore, create a list of all the things in your day that you *need* versus what you *want*. Make it clear to yourself that if you don't need it, but you want it, then you can't have it unless you follow through with healthy lifestyle adjustments.

Another accountability system is keeping a success jar in your home. Commit to putting some money into the jar every time you exercise. The money you put in that jar at the end of each month can go toward hiring a personal trainer, a charity, or a vacation. You pick.

Either way, choose an accountability system that motivates you to follow through with your exercise plan. Success with any goal requires follow through. As tough as it may be, your weight loss goal is completely attainable once you commit to doing the work. Being accountable for your actions is a great learning opportunity. You must make your weight loss journey your highest priority for it to manifest into reality. Create an accountability system that gets you to do it.

Track your days in the gym and hold yourself accountable each week. The goal is to love the feeling of being active. See yourself over that sedentary hump so that you can understand what being fit really means.

EXERCISES

(1) What type of accountability system will I adopt?

(2) What are the things I need versus want each day?

(3) How will I ensure that I show up to each scheduled exercise day?

(4) What is my weekly activity goal?

TOOL 34. HIRE A PERSONAL TRAINER

Call me biased, since I'm a personal trainer myself, but even trainers have trainers. Yup, that's true. I have friends who compete in figure competitions (shout out to Hedda Royce from www.g-loves.com), and they hire coaches to train them for competition. There's a huge accountability factor when you hire a trainer.

Nowadays, personal training has become a very sophisticated industry, and more trainers are achieving a higher level of education. Trainers don't assess or treat injuries, but trainer courses do teach injury prevention. Some workshops focus on improving functional movement, for daily movements such as lifting, pulling, pushing, and bending. Trainers also teach proper biomechanics which means having correct form during all movement.

Trainers can:

- provide basic nutrition tips;

- watch your form as you exercise;

- teach you new exercises;

- write out new workouts so that you never plateau;

- improve your sporting skills and get you stronger, more balanced, leaner, and faster; and

- hold you accountable so that you show up to the gym.

It's good to hire a trainer who has strong referrals. There are so many trainers out there, and it can be challenging to find the best one for you. Ask your friends, coworkers, or anyone you trust about their trainer. Find out what the trainer's credentials are and what makes him or her great. Determine if the trainer's background fits your needs. You can also scout out trainers at local health clubs by watching what they do with their clients. Look for their attentiveness, program design, personality, and interaction with their clients. Do they appear to possess the right skills for your success? Do they look focused, and are they watching their client's form? Try a trainer out for a session, and then commit if he or she meets your expectations. Don't fear the unknown of not clicking with a trainer. After all, you're not marrying them!

You might find the gym to be an intimidating place with new state of the art equipment and devices that you've never seen before and have no idea how to use. This is a very normal reaction. Great news! Most gyms provide you with a free personal training session to help you learn the functions of each machine. After this complimentary session is used, you may want to continue on with that trainer. A good trainer knows exactly what you need to do in the gym. For example, I have a client who is a surgeon, and on certain days he arrives to the session with stiff, tight muscles that don't allow him to move well. On these days, I emphasize stretching and functional movements that hone in on posture and proper breathing techniques. The sessions are always challenging for him because we're "undoing" the disastrous posture he's been in all day. A good trainer will know what a client needs the second he or she arrives. Great trainers always get their clients feeling much better when they leave compared to when they first walked in.

If you simply don't have the funds to hire a trainer full time, consider hiring a trainer every four weeks. Ask the trainer to build you an individualized program. He or she can base your program on your postural assessments, fitness history, injury history, and any physical limitations you have.

Make sure the trainer understands your goals and walks you through the program so that you can make the most out of your gym experience on your own.

Choose a trainer you can relate to and whose knowledge is up-to-date. Ask about their credentials. Make sure your trainer is currently CPR/AED/first-aid certified and also insured. The top two degrees for training are kinesiology and exercise physiology. Some notable certifications include ACSM, NASM, ACE, NSCA, Pilates, and yoga.

The cost of a good trainer varies from state to state. Trainers have a twenty-four-hour cancellation policy that forces you to show up; otherwise, you're charged for the session. If this doesn't motivate you to show up, I'm not sure what will. It always makes me laugh when this policy upsets people because in all actuality, it accomplishes the overall intention—that is, to get you into the gym and hold you accountable.

EXERCISES

(1) Where do I want to train (home or gym)?

(2) How was my experience with a trainer?

(3) What do I expect from my training experience? (Be specific.)

TOOL 35. VISIT A CHIROPRACTOR, MASSEUSE, OR ACUPUNCTURIST

Your body needs alignment and balance. Chiropractic, massage, and acupuncture do just that. If you lead a stressful life then you won't be successful at losing weight. Just like your mind needs to relax, so does your body.

Let's start with chiropractic care, my favorite. Chiropractic care is an art, science, and philosophy that frees up the nervous system from interference. Chiropractic adjustments enable your body to live up to its full potential again by restoring motion to it after a sedentary day. It also corrects vertebral subluxations (misalignment of the spine) that cause neurological interference. Subluxations negatively affect every system in the body. If you're tight or have issues such as poor digestion, circulatory issues, orthopedic issues, headaches, or chronic stiffness and pain, then visit a chiropractor. Chronic stiffness and poor posture may be to blame for your exhaustion each day, too. Chiropractic care can also accelerate your recovery time from an injury.

Massages complement chiropractic care. Massage focuses on the soft tissues. There are many types of massage including deep tissue, Swedish, Thai, hot stone, or trigger-point massage. Make sure you stretch your muscles after your massage to help restore the muscle's correct positioning in the body. It's up to you to be conscious of what this feels like. Ask your chiropractor to demonstrate what an optimal posture looks like, using your body as the example. Simply have him or her realign how your movement and posture should flow each day so that you can begin working on this at home and at work. Make sure you do it.

Acupuncture also accelerates the recovery process by sending fresh blood and endorphins to an injury. Acupuncture opens up the body's meridian points by freeing up any stagnant energy. When your chakras or energy in the body is trapped, your body releases stress hormones such as norepinephrine and cortisol. Keeping your body relaxed prevents these hormones from circulating. Because acupuncture relaxes the body, it's highly recommended for people who lead stressful lives.

Chiropractic care, massage, and acupuncture can prevent injury and disease. If I sit for long periods of time and my neck gets stiff, then I get a chiropractic adjustment. JZ instantly returns! Some days I get a massage. I get acupuncture if I'm injured. Some chiropractic offices house all three therapies for your convenience.

Treat your body well. Chiropractic care, massage therapy, and acupuncture help your body operate like a finely tuned machine. I've personally used all three of these specialties to completely overcome back issues I've contended with from car accidents over the years. What an awesome recovery. Alternative healing is amazing and should be seriously considered each month. Open your mind to it.

EXERCISES

(1) Where do I experience muscular/skeletal pain or discomfort?

(2) When is my first treatment scheduled?

(3) What was my experience like?

TOOL 36. DRAIN YOUR LYMPHATIC SYSTEM

Being overweight puts you at risk for many physiological and physical complications. You're more sensitive to food, your gastrointestinal tract isn't optimal, your heart and arteries may be diseased, and you might be prediabetic or prone to cancer and not even know it. Not to scare you, but this is why you must decide to do something about your weight today. Keep your lymphatic system stimulated!

The lymphatic system absorbs and transports your fatty acids, fat, and chyle from the circulatory system. It also aids in the transport of white blood cells both to and from the lymph nodes into the bones. This helps strengthen your immune system. Can you imagine shaking up your lymphatic system just so you can decrease your incidences of illness while mobilizing fat out of your cells? How cool is that? Walking around all day long with stress in your body traps vicious byproducts in your muscles and organs, especially when you remain sedentary. Kangoo jumps, a mini trampoline, the Power Plate, or any other device that shakes up your lymphatic system helps you eliminate the waste from your body's tissues. I love taking my friend Jayne Justice's Kangoo classes on the Manhattan Beach pier on Saturday mornings. I leave her class feeling euphoric. Raj Donald of Indiana and Mario Godiva Green of New York City are two more well respected Kangoo masters. If you ever have the opportunity to take a class with any of them, consider yourself lucky.

I have my seventy-three-year-old client jumping on a mini trampoline. He loves it. Anyone can do it no matter how old or overweight you are. With proper execution, you get the full benefit of stimulating lymphatic drainage while getting cardiovascular exercise. Get rid of your fear of trying something new. Try one of these new exercise gadgets, and see some great progress toward your goal.

EXERCISES

(1) Where can I Kangoo, bounce on a trampoline or use a Power Plate?

(2) What was my first experience with one of these gadgets like?

(3) On average, how often do I get sick each year?

(4) How does lymphatic drainage improve my immune system?

TOOL 37. DO A CLEANSE

A healthy gut is one of the most important aspects of optimal health. Your gastrointestinal (GI) tract has different parts, all of which play a different role in digestion and in the assimilation of nutrients. The GI tract breaks down food at the mouth, digests food in the stomach, absorbs the molecules of digestion, assimilates the nutrients from food in the small intestine, and eliminates the body's nonessential molecules through the colon. This entire process creates water as a byproduct. If this process is in any way compromised, then mental and physical disease can occur.

When you don't provide your gut with the right foods, your GI tract can't perform well. By replacing suboptimal, processed food with organic food, you get a healthier gut. This strengthens the gut's ability to assimilate molecules to the cells in the body. You may have been eating poorly for years. Years of aspartame and phosphoric acid consumption from diet sodas, hydrogenated oil found in potato chips and brownie mixes, and low-grade supplements can mess up your gut, too. If you suffer from constipation, diarrhea, gas, bloating, pain, or food allergies, then your GI tract is crying for help every day. Start listening to it! Eliminate the food sources that cause GI distress. Start adding in the foods that your body needs including five servings of vegetables, particularly dark green leafy ones, fibrous fruits (apples, berries, peaches, pears, plums), and lean proteins. Fermented vegetables (pickles and sauerkraut) are excellent for promoting the growth of healthy flora in the intestinal wall. This contributes to the effective digestibility of all vegetables in the intestines.

Consider how quickly you consume your food. Do you fully chew your food, or are you a speed racer when you eat? How many times do you put your fork down in between bites? No meal should be consumed in less than ten minutes. Please understand how important this is: Say you have a coworker you rely on for a certain task, but he fails to get it done. When his performance lacks completion and it falls back on you, you get exhausted and can't perform your own tasks well because you're busy picking up his slack. Don't you hate that? This happens in your GI tract when you don't chew your food up well. Your GI tract may fail to break down the food particles in your gut because you didn't chew enough. This causes other parts of the tract to work overtime. The result may be poor food particle assimilation in the lower gut because the upper gut slacked off like that coworker did. This will lead to sensitivities in the gut. You must therefore chew your food up.

Years ago, cleansing was used as a method to alleviate bacterial infections before antiobiotics were discovered. Nowadays, cleanses are used to improve one's body composition and digestive health which contribute to higher energy levels. Restoring proper gut health can be accomplished through the right cleanse or a combination of different cleanses. The most popular one is the colon cleanse, since everything in the body relies heavily on the colon.

A colon cleanse can:

- remove excess stool and nonspecific toxins from the intestinal tract and the colon;

- flush out your kidneys and digestive tract;

- purify your cells and lymphatic system;

- eliminate unusable waste that builds up in the joints and muscles;

- relieve pressure on your nerves, vessels, and arteries;

- keep your skin vibrant;

- keep your bloodstream healthy; and

- diminish sugar cravings.

Other cleanses exist but it's important to find the right one for you. Make sure you work with a professional who knows what they're doing. Cleansing the colon is universal. Cleansing other systems is where the individuality comes in. My friend Jayne Justice does a very basic food-based cleanse with her clients. This cleanse is excellent for beginners. She teaches people how to be hypersensitive to their fruit and vegetable intake each day. During her seven day cleanse, I only consumed vegetables, fibrous fruits, lots of water and a special mixture designed to help clean my colon. As a result, I felt lighter and I realized that I wasn't consuming enough vegetables prior to the cleanse. Those were two benefits that I received from doing her cleanse. For a more in depth cleanse that involves products, work with medical experts such as Garry Gordon, M.D. in Arizona or Mark Hyman, M.D. in Massachusetts. Work with a specialist who has the experience to determine which cleanse is right for you based on your signs and symptoms.

To compliment any cleanse, you should consider either colonics or enemas. I work directly with a colonics specialist, Georgette Grabenhorst in California, who is a genius at eliminating any unwanted bacteria and reestablishing healthy levels of good bacteria in your intestines. Between her and Jayne, I call their approach my "California Experience," and it's available to anyone nationwide. Contact me by email at jz@jzfitness.com. Georgette once told me that an unhealthy gut is like looking through dirty windows. You can see through them, but you can't see everything clearly.

Speak with your doctor first. If you wish to stay in your local area for such services, then consider contacting a local gastroenterologist who can refer you to a qualified nutritionist and reputable colonics center. Gastrointestinal health is one of the most powerful tools in your weight-loss journey. A healthy gut is a healthy body.

EXERCISES

(1) Who are the cleansing specialists in my area?

(2) How often do I have good bowel movements?

(3) Do I experience stomach irritation on a regular basis? If so, have I ever checked for any food sensitivities?

TOOL 38. JUST BREATHE

We live in a very fast-paced society that requires us to go, go, go. As a result, we gain tension in our bodies, shortness of breath, acidity in the blood, and high levels of anxiety. Your body is not built for these conditions on a chronic basis. The body needs inner peace. Inner peace is established from a state of equilibrium. You remember the word *homeostasis* from fifth grade? That's what your body strives for every day. Being out of homeostasis stimulates your stress hormones again, which resonates in your muscles, organs, and entire being. You'll feel nervous, jittery, anxious, unrested at night, physically and mentally exhausted, and perhaps emotionally unstable. Feeling this way causes you to be unproductive, moody, tired, irritable, and quite impatient with the world around you. This causes you to overeat.

The most efficient way to keep calm throughout your day is to practice deep pelvic breathing. Start off by inhaling through your nose, and sealing that breath of newness for a moment before releasing it through your mouth on the exhale. Continue with deep breaths in and out through your nose with your mouth closed. Allow your breath to sound like ocean waves hitting the shore.

Use this tool every day. Don't wait. Let's put this into practice. When you have a deadline and the clock is ticking to the end, deep breathing exercises are great for your mind and body. My love for yoga (tool 6) falls in alignment with this methodology. Yoga classes teach you excellent breathing exercises. Incorporate these breathing exercises into your everyday activities: work, school, relationships, personal experiences, and everything else that throws your body out of homeostasis.

When is the best time to perform these breathing exercises? Always. Below are several opportunities to utilize your deep breathing exercises to help improve your day:

- When you're under a lot of stress at work

- When you're sitting in traffic

- When you're waiting in a long line

- When you're in an argument

- When you're about to make a speech

- When you're in a debate

- When you're attempting to go the bathroom

- When you're attempting to go to sleep

- When you're exercising

- When you're in pain

- When you're nervous

This is a very important tool for virtually everyone, yet it's usually underutilized. During your weight-loss journey, you should experience love, laughter, and light in your life. If darkness sweeps the ground beneath you and covers your day with negative energy, then it's truly up to you to step into the light of happiness and become one with your peace of mind again. Don't allow anything to consume your mind with stressful thoughts. You deserve to feel like you're on top of the world by fueling your body with positive energy. The easiest and most tangible way of getting there is learning how to breathe deeply when your body needs to settle down or when you just need to take a moment for yourself again.

EXERCISES

1) Cover your right nostril and slowly inhale for four counts by allowing the air to enter in from the bottom of the belly, working its way up through the chest and into the nostril. Seal the breath at the top by holding both nostrils. Then release your finger on the right nostril and cover the left nostril and slowly exhale for four counts. Inhale through that same nostril for four counts and then exhale through the opposite nostril for four counts. Keep repeating this for one minute.

2) Lie down on the floor or in bed. Close your eyes. Focus on breathing into the lower abdomen, rather

> than into your chest. Inhale through your nose for four counts and slowly exhale through pursed lips for four counts. Repeat this ten times or for as long as you wish.

TOOL 39. GO TO A THEME PARK

People have told me that they get a lot more movement at a theme park than they do in a typical day. The steps they took in that single day sometimes exceed what they've done in three days. This is understandable. When you go to a massive place like a park, you move a lot from one attraction to the next.

The only culprit in theme parks is that the food is usually quite unhealthy. So, what do you do? Follow these easy tips:

1) Go to the park having already eaten.

2) Pack healthy snacks.

3) Choose protein for your meals and snacks. A burger or chicken breast beats those chili fries, cotton candy, and spare ribs you may have eaten in the past. It's okay that these proteins aren't grass-fed beef or free-range organic chicken. As long as your portions are correct, you'll be ahead of most theme park attendees.

One way to manage temptation at a park is to not even entertain the thought of junk food, no matter what. Don't state, "I could really go for a funnel cake or a plate of chicken wings and french fries." Spare yourself from the fat, carbs, and calories. Eating that type of food is like putting diesel fuel into a Honda. You just don't do it. Thinking this way causes you to choose food with a conscious mind.

So why are we so addicted to all that stuff, then? Theme park food cravings can stem from childhood from when your parents fed you this stuff. It also aligns with all other food addictions you have. If you have children, it's up to you to break that cycle. Teach your children healthy behaviors. It's okay to feed your child with an ice cream cone or a pretzel, but keep their other meals healthy. Also realize that theme park food will sidetrack you from your goal. Is it worth it? Just realize that fatty, processed food will diminish your energy and your ability to walk around all day. Realize that your family and/or friends deserve good company. Junk food will cause your body to drag and your stomach to hurt. Eating healthy will allow you to power through the theme park. Use self-talk when you're standing in line for lunch and tell yourself, "I will only order food that's healthy and that will help keep my energy levels up for the day!"

Keep your theme park experience active by considering the following activities:

- Since much of your time will be spent on lines waiting for the rides, plan on sprinting from ride to ride. Race against your family members.

- Choose one ride in each section of the park, and bounce around each section so that you walk more and increase your steps that day.

- Put together a scavenger hunt with the members of your group. For example, come up with two teams who go on rides together. Each team should experience ten rides and get a signature from the operators of each ride. You might even consider adding the challenge of doing twenty five jumping jacks, push-ups, or squats in front of the operator at each ride to qualify your team for each signature.

Have fun! You have the power to be in control of your behaviors while showing your company an amazing time.

EXERCISES

(1) What do I normally love to eat at theme parks?

(2) What did I choose to eat at the theme park this time?

(3) Which game(s) did we play?

TOOL 40. CHOOSE A MARTIAL ARTS DISCIPLINE

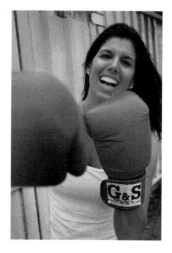

Learning about discipline and commitment are two areas you master through martial arts. This can be your initiation to a healthier way of life. Martial arts focuses on flexibility, centeredness, and endurance. When you're centered and generate the right energy from the right places in your body, you deepen your *qigong*

(breath), increase mental awareness, and tap into your spiritual side. Martial arts also helps you feel empowered to achieve virtually anything.

Talk about burning a ton of calories and working your core muscles! Whew—martial arts does just that. There are many disciplines to choose from, so first see what you have access to. Learn about each one, and see which one fits your personality and fitness capabilities. If you suffer from any major orthopedic or cardiorespiratory conditions, then consult your doctor first.

Here's a list of martial arts to choose from:

- Tai Chi: slow and meditative energy movement. Focus: relaxation and balance.

- Karate: sharp blows and kicks. Focus: indigenous fighting.

- Krav Maga: a combination of wrestling, grappling, and striking. Focus: contact fighting.

- Taekwando: similar to karate. Focus: elaborate kicking.

- Capoeira: a combination of martial arts, music, and dance. Focus: trickery.

- Brazilian Jujitsu: grappling and ground fighting. Focus: combat.

Even though boxing is not considered a martial art, I personally love it because I grew up around boxing. My grandfather, Izzy Zerling, started G & S Sporting Goods in New York City (www.gsboxing.com) back in 1937. His entire life was one big fight. He migrated to America at the age of eleven years old. He worked at a young age to support his mother since he lost his father at the age of two. He became an amateur fighter at the age of sixteen, but due to a heart murmur couldn't enter the Golden Gloves Tournament! He turned pro in 1932 and fought admirably for five years before opening up G & S on the Lower East Side to teach youngsters the art of self-defense and take the gangs off the street! It gave youngsters a place to vent some of their anger through an appropriate outlet. He taught teenagers the value of education and encouraged them to keep their grades at a respectable level. The symbolism of fighting throughout my grandfather's life is epic to everyone who knew him. My grandfather's determination kept him alive until his mid nineties. G&S symbolizes more than just the best boxing gear out there. It truly reflects how determination can elevate individuals to high altitudes of success.

All martial arts empower you to tap into your own source of independence and charisma. Martial arts can help you find the bright light within you that shines toward your success. No one and nothing can ever dim that light within you! If you need that extra fight in you, then consider enrolling in martial arts.

EXERCISES

(1) Which martial arts discipline appeals to me?

(2) What are my two fears about taking martial arts? How can I overcome them?

(3) What are the types of martial arts or boxing programs offered in my town?

TOOL 41. SIGN UP FOR A RACE

Signing up for a 5K (3.1 miles) or a 10K (6.2 miles) doesn't mean that you have to compete to win. Rather, it gives you a goal to train toward. Every time you feel like you hit a plateau and your workouts aren't challenging enough, sign up for a race and take your training to the next level. I know that Nike hosts a running club for beginners and intermediate runners who wish to train. You get to meet new people, improve your cardiovascular fitness level, and develop good running skills in groups. You will feel challenged at first, but you will improve. Group settings help facilitate the appropriate level of training, intensity, distance, and a strong commitment from you. Some people choose to train alone or run with a partner.

Below are some helpful tips to get you started:

- Get the right shoes.

- Be well hydrated.

- Stretch your calves, hips, quads, and hamstrings well before you run.

- Determine what a 5K is by outlining a path that you wish to walk and/or run.

- Start with a walk, and in time, move to a jog and then a run.

The speed of your run doesn't matter unless your goal is to cover a distance in a certain period of time. Just to give you an idea, you're looking at a thirty-minute to one hour commitment depending on how fast you go. If you are completely out of shape and walking is a challenge for you, then start there. The first week will be all about establishing the distance and the time it took you to complete the 5K distance. You'll reassess your level of physical activity each week. Consider doing intervals (tool 43) at some point throughout the course of training.

Walking slowly every day for weeks at a time won't build up your cardiovascular fitness level. The goal is to exert enough effort so that you can't hold a conversation with someone, but not to where you're barely breathing.

Consider hiring a trainer to guide you through the preparation of running a race. My friend Jason Karp is a running coach who has written many books on running that are useful for both athletes and non-athletes. Consider reading them and finding a running coach near you for training. Use a heart-rate monitor so that you can train in your heart-rate zone (Polar heart rate monitors are great). The VO_2 max test (tool 42) helps you determine your heart rate zones. If you can't access this test in the beginning, don't worry about it. Focus on challenging yourself one day at a time. Make your training fun by downloading good music to listen to that'll pump you up. Also try new routes to avoid monotony.

You don't have to run a mile all at once. You don't need to cover a 3.1-mile distance all at once either. Increase your distance over time. Improve your progress each time you train. Set specific goals for yourself. For example, go around your block once, then twice, three times, and so on until you complete a mile. From there, do a mile and a half. Next, increase your distance to two miles, and so on. A 5K is a great start and isn't hard to do once you do it.

If the thought of signing up for a 5K is too overwhelming for you, then schedule your 5K in six months from now. This will leave you plenty of time to train.

A great story: A woman that I work with decided to run a marathon, which prompted her to lose eighty-three pounds. She weighed 250 pounds at the time. By the time the marathon rolled around, she had dropped thirty pounds and ran at 220 pounds. As hard as this was, she did it. The marathon created an urgency to lose weight. Afterward, she continued her weight-loss journey until reaching her current weight of 167 pounds, and she's aiming for lower. She's more active now than ever before. She officially graduated from the mindset of being an overweight individual. She claims that life is ten times better at her current lean weight and that nothing tastes good enough for her to compromise her new lifestyle. She knows that her past lifestyle caused her to be fat so she had to dump that lifestyle forever. She is fully committed. She's a great example of someone who took this tool and followed through with it even though she had to battle the barriers of saboteurs and other hiccups along the way. I was shocked when she told me that people who've known her for years don't compliment her new body. But she decided that as long as she's happy, that's all that's important. Smart girl.

Anything is possible. Get rid of any doubts and any barriers. Be great for yourself! Train for a race because you can!

EXERCISES

(1) Which 5K race in my town will I sign up for?

(2) How will I start my training?

(3) Whom can I run with each week? (Alone is okay.)

TOOL 42. TEST YOUR FITNESS LEVELS

Having a starting point allows you to see how training improves your fitness levels. Improving your fitness levels through the correct training program is important. Measuring your fitness levels will motivate you to work out with a plan of action rather than simply going through the motions of working out. It's far more rewarding to work out with intentions compared to simply showing up at the gym with no plan in mind. Don't worry so much about where you start from because you can only get better. The important factor is to improve your own performance. Learn how to compete against your own scores and appreciate your own personal growth. Don't compare yourself to others.

Not every place offers every fitness test. Of the ones listed below, strive to get a VO_2 max test since it's the best indicator for determining your cardiovascular fitness level.

VO_2 max is the volume of oxygen in milliliters per kilogram of body weight per minute that your cardiorespiratory system can push to the cells in your body during exercise. The higher your score is, the more fit you are. The great thing about the VO_2 max test is that it tells you how many miles per gallon your body gets, rhetorically speaking. Body fat and excess weight lower your VO_2 score. When you lose weight, your VO_2 score improves. Your VO_2 max score is also improved through interval training (tool 43) and proper nutrition.

The VO_2 max test is usually performed on a bike or treadmill. Whatever you plan to do more of will determine which equipment you should be tested on. In other words, if you're a runner, then perform your test on the treadmill over the bicycle. Your score between the bike and the treadmill can be different.

Some places where you can get your fitness levels tested include the following:

- A local health club
- A personal trainer's facility
- Sports-performance clinics
- Physical-therapy clinics
- A local university

These are some tests to consider:

- VO_2 max test
- Push-up test
- Crunch assessment

- Isometric dynamometry

- Sit-and-reach test

- Pull-ups or hanging chin holds

- Body composition

- One-mile run

For a little friendly competition, organize a contest between your friends. Consider organizing teams in training to see which team can improve their VO_2 max score the most. Also consider organizing a push-up contest to see who can perform the most push-ups and who can hold the longest planks (when you are positioned on your forearms and toes). Organize a weight-loss competition, too. Set up some sort of reward system for the winners. It can be monetary, a gift certificate somewhere, or a fitness device (new treadmill, bike, heart-rate monitor, etc.). Make the competition fun.

EXERCISES

(1) Which facilities around me offer these tests?

(2) When can I test my fitness levels?

(3) What are my VO_2 max score and target heart rate zone?

TOOL 43. PERFORM INTERVAL TRAINING

Interval training rocks the socks off of any other cardiovascular program I know of. It improves your cardiovascular fitness levels (VO$_2$ max values), lactate threshold, natural production and release of growth hormone, fat burning, and the utilization of excess blood sugar. Interval training can also improve your sex life, and it increases your caloric expense even after you're done training. Can you imagine exercising at high intensities for only thirty to forty minutes at a time and burning a boatload of calories? Now that's what I'm talking about!

What is interval training? I like to describe it as cardiovascular exercise that works your cardio (heart) respiratory (lungs) systems through a full range of motion. You know how you extend and flex your arm through a full range of motion during a bicep curl? You do this so that your entire biceps muscle gets stronger. The same goes for when you train your cardiorespiratory systems. You want to train them through a full range of motion by challenging the systems both aerobically (with oxygen) and anaerobically (without oxygen) on a cellular level. The way to do this is through elevating your heart rate to high rates and then decreasing the level immediately following the high-intensity sprint. The harder the activity, the higher your heart rate will go. The easier the activity, the lower your heart rate is. Interval training is working both anaerobically (during the high-intensity bouts that spike your heart rate due to an increase in speed and/or resistance) and aerobically (when your heart rate and the work intensity decrease, allowing your body to use a higher percentage of oxygen for energy). This cycle actually improves the strength of your heart muscle and increases your stroke volume, the volume of blood that your ventricle pushes out of your heart with each beat to all the cells in the body. Improving your stroke volume will increase the amount of nutrients, oxygen, and other goodies that go to your body.

Even though interval training may sound intimidating, it's one of the best ways to improve your cardiorespiratory fitness level. Take, for example, a person living in New York City who catches buses and cabs all day long. This action requires excellent cardiorespiratory fitness. When I lived in New York City, I had to sprint up the block like a bolt of lightning to catch a bus. I never knew when the next bus would come. I avoided a twenty-minute wait by doing this.

Think of a time when movement caused you to lose your breath. Think of the time when you couldn't keep up with others because they were moving too quickly for you. Think of the time when you were intimate with your partner and got dizzy. Interval training allows your body to improve in all these areas. Your body will eventually adapt to some of the most challenging stimuli in your everyday life. These experiences will eventually get much easier for you.

Intervals do not have to be hard-core to start. There are different interval programs you can do. First, choose the right equipment to perform your intervals on. Examples include the treadmill, a bike, an elliptical, a jump rope, or a rowing machine; other activities are swimming, hitting a heavy bag, or even performing jumping jacks in your basement. Whatever makes you happy and challenges you is great. Talk to a fitness expert about what your heart-rate zone is. Then, consider performing any of the two interval programs:

Intermediate to advanced program:

1) Warm up for five to ten minutes to prepare your muscles.

2) Sprint for one minute (all out by adding resistance and/or speed).

3) Recover for thirty seconds (back off and bring your heart rate down).

4) Repeat this five times, sprinting for one minute and recovering for thirty seconds each time.

5) After performing five intervals, recover for three to five minutes in your aerobic training zone (where you burn optimal levels of fat. You learn this value through testing your VO_2 max tool 42).

6) Repeat another round of five intervals and do so for the duration of your workout.

Beginner program:

1) Warm up for five to ten minutes to prepare your muscles.

2) Sprint for twenty seconds to your peak heart rate zone (tool 42).

3) Recover for one minute and bring your heart rate down toward your aerobic heart rate from your VO_2 max test (tool 42).

4) Repeat three times, sprinting for twenty seconds and recovering for one minute each time.

5) After three intervals, recover for five minutes in your aerobic training zone.

6) Repeat another round of three intervals with repeated sprint / recoveries.

EXERCISES

(1) What are the top two reasons why improving my cardiorespiratory fitness levels are important to me?

---

(2) Which days will I perform intervals?

---

(3) Which type of cardio exercise will I do?

TOOL 44. GET A PEDOMETER

Every adult should walk a minimum of ten thousand steps a day. There's no way of knowing how many steps you take each day without measuring with a pedometer. Getting a pedometer is a great tool to help promote more movement each day. If you're not taking at least ten thousand steps a day, then you're considered sedentary which increases your risk for heart disease, obesity, diabetes, stroke, and metabolic syndrome. So get a pedometer and start moving now. Pedometers are affordable. They are sold at most sporting-goods stores and online.

A pedometer will help you work your way up to ten thousand steps a day. Once you get it, attach it to your hip every day from the moment you rise to the moment you're ready for bed. Do not wear it in the shower, and certainly do not forget to take it off when you go to the restroom. These things are not waterproof!

Build up your progress one week at a time. For example, if you only achieve six thousand steps in your first week, don't feel defeated. Instead, improve that number by increasing your movement each day. Be happy that you now know how little you were moving before. You can change this. Increase your steps each week. It's all about working to get better, one step at a time (the pun is intended.) Don't be hard on yourself, especially in the beginning of your weight loss journey. Find gratitude for all of your accomplishments today. Just because you don't attain your initial goal, doesn't mean that you never will.

I've worked with people who get well over ten thousand steps a day. Remember, you want a *minimum* of ten thousand steps a day. If you measure thirteen thousand steps, then aim for fifteen thousand steps. The goal is to attain more movement every day no matter where you start.

Some ways to increase your steps each day include the following:

- Taking the stairs instead of the elevator
- Parking your car far from the entrance of wherever you go
- Walking to the store versus driving
- Walking around the entire grocery store versus just going down the aisles you need to visit
- Taking a morning and/or evening walk

- Getting up from your desk and walking around your house and/or office

- Playing with your pet for ten minutes a day

- Doing household chores every day

- Putting the shopping cart back instead of leaving it out, which can dent another car anyway

- Wearing the right walking shoes (tool 55) and briskly walking through the largest mall around you

I'll never forget the time my fiancé and I went to Universal Studios in Southern California. We ended up taking four tremendous escalators all the way down from the top of the park to the Jurassic Park ride down below. Afterward, when we headed back up, there was a huge crowd of people taking the escalators, and I looked at Alan as if to say, "We're climbing the stairs." He asked, "Are you serious, honey?" And I was. Together we walked up three out of four flights of stairs. Universal told me that there are 379 stairs from top to bottom. If you divide that by three, assuming that they're equally distributed, Alan and I walked up 252 stairs. Awesome, right? Try it yourself.

Once you purchase a pedometer and wear it, you'll learn fun ways to increase your step count each day. Look for every opportunity you can. Just promise yourself that you'll reflect on where you're coming from as you increase your steps each day. You owe it to yourself to feel good about what you've done rather than what you feel like you need to do. Be patient with yourself. You will get better with consistency!

EXERCISES

(1) How many steps did I take on my first day according to my pedometer?

(2) How will I improve the number of steps I take tomorrow?

TOOL 45. TAKE A DANCE CLASS

Historically, dance told stories and was considered a ritual or scare tactic against those who threatened a village. Today, dance is used to celebrate, express oneself, and burn calories. The only time dance is used as a scare tactic is when a person has two left feet and brings in eighties dance moves again. I couldn't resist being silly. If you throw away your inhibitions and just let yourself go, you'll find the light within yourself when you dance. When I was growing up, my mother used to put on some of her favorite records (remember those?), and we danced in the living room all morning long. We sang songs together and acted silly. I remember sweating and my heart pounding. My brother and I would dance like wild children and collapse to the floor in laughter.

Dancing promotes weight loss since it works major muscle groups and raises your heart rate, thereby burning lots of calories. Music truly awakens your soul. It's fun and it really pumps you up.

There are different types of dance classes to choose from:

- Zumba
- Belly dancing
- Pole dancing
- Salsa
- Country line dancing
- Jazz
- Tap
- Ballet
- Hip-hop

Dancing connects your conscious state of mind with your heart. It's all about self-expression, which can boost your mood, too. There are many upbeat and easy-to-learn dance classes out there, and plenty of caring instructors, so trust that you'll find one that you love. I love taking the vivacious and adorable Melissa Zugell's Zumba class and the hot, spicy Lisa Nunziella's salsa class at Gold's Gym in Venice. You will find your favorites, too.

Moving your body continuously increases your cardiorespiratory fitness levels. Dancing also allows you to rediscover your sexiness. Do you know that when you dance at a high intensity for an hour straight, you can easily burn five hundred calories?

If you're shy, this is a phenomenal out-of–the-box tool to help open you up. I am a big believer in addressing your introverted side through dancing. Dance helps you to explore your inner appeal and unpeel your layers of protection. Work through your shyness because nowadays, dance classes are a huge trend in gyms. Modern-day dance classes attract virtually anyone of any size, age group, and skill set. So enjoy an awesome workout to great music.

Dance in your own home and even in your car. Music acts like a bookmark in life since it reminds us of where we were when the songs came out. I was listening to Macho Man in my car the other day, and I was automatically brought back to my childhood. I started to dance in my car. Neighboring cars thought I was nuts, but heck, I was having fun!

I remember when I worked for the Henry Street Playhouse in New York City. I directed a children's show titled *Children Just Like Me.* As the director, I decided to make one of the rehearsals a musical journey to touch children's hearts in a spontaneous way. I played different genres of music, and the children embodied each song with different movements that revealed their interpretation. I was amazed by how naturally the kids responded to this exercise. Some of them danced; some of them cried. The kids who appeared uncomfortable still engaged in some way. That must have been one of the most powerful workshops I've ever conducted.

Find the power within you and take a dance class. It's time to get in touch with the arts again.

EXERCISES

(1) Which type of dance class interests me?

(2) Which music did I dance to this week, and what did it remind me of?

(3) Did I feel shy, or did I embrace it?

TOOL 46. DO FIFTY TO ONE HUNDRED CRUNCHES A DAY

Crunches allow you to be in tuned with your trunk. This is your entire upper body from your hips to your chin. It houses all of your vital organs. When you feel your abs working, you'll want to treat them right. If your belly is full of junk food, you'll be too nauseated to follow through with this tool. You'll therefore want to limit the stuffed feeling by eating healthy food so you can move your trunk more. Some people don't like this tool if their belly is too big because it's uncomfortable. This is exactly why this tool is perfect. It provides you urgency to lose the belly fat. If you can't do a crunch, can you imagine how your organs feel while doing their jobs?

Start with twenty-five crunches. Then add on twenty-five each week. Do fifty to a hundred eventually. Never do crunches when you're too sore. Keep in mind that the discomfort you're feeling may only be temporary from being overweight. If you experience any lower back pain or have any sort of spinal injuries, then I don't advise you use this tool unless you get clearance from your doctor.

An alternative to crunches are plank which are held isometrically (with no movement). Consider doing five sets. Hold each set for ten to twenty seconds. Nothing should exacerbate any orthopedic condition. Avoid isometric activity if you have high blood pressure. For those of you who want to try out planks, here's how you do them. First, get on your hands and knees. Next, go onto your forearms and position them parallel to one another. Position your chest in between your elbows. Then, extend one foot out at a time and get onto your toes. You are essentially balancing on your forearms and toes. Make sure you're squeezing your abdominals very tight. Think of pulling your belly button up and in toward your spine. Breathe. Some plank variations include lifting one arm up and balancing on three limbs for ten seconds, switching to the other arm, lifting one leg up at a time, and even lifting the opposite arm and leg up simultaneously. These variations make the plank far more challenging.

It's best to warm up your back muscles before performing crunches. Consider a few sun salutations (a yoga move) to warm up your spine, core, and lower body. When performing crunches, make sure you always draw your belly button up and in toward your spine. This is called abdominal bracing and will protect your lower back from overextending. One way to know that you're bracing your core muscles is to lie on your back and place your hands under your lower back, feeling the curvature of your back flattening into the ground into your hands.

Below is a sample workout:

- Twenty-five standard crunches with hands underneath your occipital lobe (hands cradling the neck)

- Fifty bicycle crunches (on your back, you will cradle your neck with your hands and bring your legs up to ninety degrees. Extend one leg out at a time and have the opposite elbow touch the bending knee. Alternate between sides.)

- Twenty-five reverse crunches with hands next to the lower back

EXERCISES

(1) Do I have any backaches that I must discuss with my doctor?

(2) How many crunches did I perform today?

(3) What food did I avoid eating today due to performing crunches?

TOOL 47. STRETCH EVERY DAY

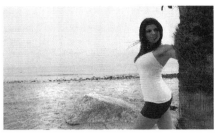

As human beings, we're not built to sit. So many people sit at a desk all day long. This is a physiological and physical disaster waiting to happen. You should not be seated in one position for more than thirty minutes at a time. I don't care how much work you have or how many deadlines you must meet. If you sit all day then you develop poor posture, which will domino into poor circulation, a decrease in natural hormone production, a diminished metabolism, chronic joint pain, and an increased risk of osteoporosis. Experiencing pain and discomfort on a daily basis will keep you unmotivated to go to the gym. No one likes physical discomfort during a workout. Therefore, keep your body limber every day.

Stretching alleviates physical complications before they happen. Stretching also allows proper blood flow to your joints and muscles. Motion reduces gravitational pull on your spine. A body without proper circulation gets tired and tight. You'll even shrink an inch or two from sitting a lot because the vertebral spaces in your spine shorten due to gravitational pull. This will eventually cause back pain, stenosis, sciatica, hip pain, other joint pain, and lots of muscle tightness. Therefore, keep your sedentary behaviors to a minimum.

If you laid on your couch all day yesterday watching television, then you must get off your butt today and do something active. Your body will slowly deteriorate if you remain sedentary. Many people who work desk jobs are considered sedentary, but sedentary behaviors are seen in other areas of life, too. Take a moment to see if this is you. How long do you sit at work, if you had to guess? How long is your commute to work? How many hours a day do you watch television? How many meetings do you sit through? Did you travel today? Did you sit in the waiting room for an appointment? Add up all those hours. You'll be shocked! This is why you must stretch!

Stretch many times a day, every single day. Stretch on the hour every hour so that you remember to do so. Stretch against the wall, at your desk, using a stability ball and maybe a foam roller. Stretch while you're talking to a client on the phone. Believe it or not, standing will increase your energy through the phone, which may be more effective for you anyway. Try it. Below are common postural issues and stretches to add to your day. Many of these stretches may appear unfamiliar to you. I recommend that you look them up on Google or YouTube for proper demonstration. You may also ask a local personal trainer to lead you through a stretching session. These stretches will help address any muscle imbalances you have when performed consistently and correctly.

Issue	Stretch
Forward shoulders	Chest stretch using a doorway
Tight lower back	Supine piriformis stretch
Tight lower back	Standing hamstring stretch
Tight calves	Wall stretch
Tight shoulders	Wall stretch latissimus dorsi
Tight shoulders	Forward fold with hands clasped in back
Tight neck	Lateral flexion and forward flexion of neck

EXERCISES

(1) How many hours do I sit a day?

(2) Which stretches will I perform each hour? (Pick three a day to do every hour and hold each stretch for at least thirty seconds.)

(3) How many times did I stretch today?

TOOL 48. GET A GREAT BED

I mentioned in tool 29 that good-quality sleep is paramount for successful weight loss. I speak with so many people who don't sleep well, and most of them are overweight. I can honestly say that I didn't always sleep well myself. For me, my bed was to blame. I didn't have a horrible bed, but when I purchased my California king Tempur-Pedic bed, my whole night changed. This is by far the most comfortable bed I've ever slept in. It conforms to your body so when you sleep on your side, your shoulder isn't pushed up into your ear. When you're on your back, your spine just sinks into the foam. It feels so great on my athletic body, like I'm lying on a bed of clouds.

People who suffer from weight-control issues and joint pain can find therapeutic assistance from a good bed. It helps alleviate muscle aches and back pain. A good bed can aid in a good night's rest after a very active day. This is a great investment because six to eight hours a day are spent in bed. If you do the math, that's between 2,190 and 2,920 hours a year spent in bed. That's a lot of time. Do you now see the value in owning a great bed?

EXERCISES

(1) On average, how many hours of sleep do I get a night?

(2) How are my energy levels in the morning (0 = horrible, 5 = OK, 10 = amazing)?

(3) How old is my bed?

(4) When I wake up in the morning, how does my body physically feel?

TOOL 49. CHECK YOUR RMR

Your resting metabolic rate (RMR) is the rate at which you burn calories just by keeping your eyes open. If you were to lie awake in your bed all day without doing anything, your brain, lungs, and cardiovascular systems would still be working. The rate of work expended by all three systems combined burns a certain number of calories each day. That total number of calories represents your RMR. If these systems burn, for example, 1,200 calories alone, then how many calories do you think you should eat in order to lose weight? This is where most diets fail. And this is where most people fail at dieting. No one knows how much 1,200 calories is, and many times counting calories becomes too much of a chore.

Poor nutrition, suboptimal hormone production, excessive body fat, and a sedentary lifestyle are among some of the reasons why your RMR may not be high. A low RMR will impact your ability to burn through certain foods effectively, particularly foods that are considered high-glycemic carbohydrates (tool 68), which can hinder weight loss.

Your RMR is important to know. If you eat too few calories for too long, your body won't have enough fuel for basic life functions. Starving also steals energy from your muscles. You don't want to lose muscle. Your goal is to lose fat. If you don't feed your "engine" with enough of the right food to fuel your RMR, how do you expect to perform throughout your day? This caloric deficiency results in irritability, exhaustion, and weakness. You'll eventually quit. Starvation diets never work and never will!

Health clubs, physical-therapy offices, sports facilities, and local universities can test your RMR. One thing to remember is that you must perform this test on an empty stomach without caffeine in your system. You must also abstain from all activities that stimulate your heartbeat. A rested body will produce accurate resting results that you can depend on. Once you know your number, don't follow any diet that drops below your RMR.

After checking your RMR, ask the therapist, nutritionist, or trainer to guide you in an appropriate nutritional plan. Keep a daily journal (tool 28) and track what you're eating each day.

Focus on long-term strategies that work for you. I broke my chains of poor eating habits by utilizing many of the tools presented in this book every day of my life to this day. If one strategy doesn't work one day, pick a new one. Don't regress to your unhealthy behaviors from before. This journey can only move forward.

EXERCISES

(1) What is my RMR?

(2) What is a sensible caloric intake based on my RMR?

(3) How will I ensure that I'm eating what's right for me?

TOOL 50. TEST YOUR BODY COMPOSITION

Different types of cellular tissue are part of your body's composition, which consists of your fat mass and your fat-free mass. Your fat-free mass is everything other than fat. When you're losing weight, you want to keep the fat-free mass and lose the fat. This measurement can also allow you to determine the amount of protein you need to eat each day (tool 59).

There are different modalities for testing your body composition. The more extensive a body-composition analysis is, the more valid it is. Validity is based on the absolute value of something. Reliability is dependable but not 100 percent valid. Body mass index (BMI) is outdated because it only gives you a height-to-weight ratio and doesn't take into account how much body fat weight someone has. That is why this test is not listed below.

Don't rely solely on the scale. Remember, muscle has a metabolic advantage over fat. Visceral fat simply takes up space in the body's cavities and slows you down. Fat also sucks the oxygen out of your system, stealing it from muscle, which is why it must be reduced. Excessive body fat values also lead to heart disease.

The body composition tests out there include the following:

1. DEXA: The Dual Energy X-ray Absorptiometry Scan (DEXA) is very accurate in isolating fat, lean weight, and bone weight through X-ray. It's very valid and reliable. Most MRI imaging centers have it. The amount of radiation you receive from this scanner is minimal. This device also measures bone density for early detection of osteoporosis. You'll need a doctor's prescription for this test. The body composition printout divides the body up into different regions including the trunk, abdomen, hips, arms, and legs.

2. Hydrostatic Test: This test dunks you into water to determine fat composition. It's both valid and reliable. You get wet. Your local gym, some local colleges, and some wellness centers offer it.

3. Skin Caliper Assessment: A skin caliper test uses a special tool (calipers) to measure the skin-fold thickness of the layer of fat just under the skin at several sites on your body. Once you determine your body-fat percentage, figure out how many pounds are fat and how many pounds are fat-free mass (*Total weight* x *percent body fat = lbs. of fat. Total weight – fat lbs. = fat free lbs.*) The reliability of this test depends on who's testing you. Use the same tester every time. Virtually every health club has this assessment in their fitness department. Ask a trainer.

4. Bioelectric Impedance Analysis (BIA): This test uses electrical impedance that runs through the body and calculates the difference between fat and lean mass. It is reliable but is the least valid, depending on the model you use. This test is offered at most health clubs, or you can buy a Tanita scale for your home. Do the math to figure out what your fat-free mass is based on the body-fat percentage.

Regardless of the test you choose, stick to the same one every time you re-measure yourself. You can't compare your results between the different tests. Promise yourself that you won't get caught up in the number on the scale. When you eat well, exercise, sleep well, and manage your stress levels well, you succeed in time. Avoid comparing yourself to Joe Shmoe who lost more weight on his diet than you did. You're in two different bodies. You can always pick his brain to see how he did it. Never surrender yourself to jealousy of someone else's success. Be proud of them.

EXERCISES

(1) What is my initial body-fat percentage?

(2) Of my total weight, how much lean weight do I have?

(3) Based on tool 59, how much protein should I eat a day to equate to my lean body weight?

TOOL 51. CHECK HORMONE LEVELS

You will lose weight when you master your nutrition and exercise program. However, if you're middle aged and going through menopause or andropause, then your hormone levels might be suboptimal. It pays to check them. Hormone therapy may alter the effects of aging. Age management is the future of medicine and is a modern conversation for most people over the age of forty. From this age forward, most people begin to feel the effects of aging due to the decline in their own natural hormone production. Working in the age-management industry has taught me that suboptimal hormone levels can heavily impact metabolism, causing weight gain for inactive individuals who have poor nutritional habits. These poor habits must be conquered first.

I encourage you to get an extensive health evaluation that measures all the major hormones in the body responsible for metabolism and libido, including the following panels: thyroid stimulating hormone (TSH), T3-free, T4-free, DHEA, both total and free testosterone, dihydrotestosterone, luteinizing hormone (LH), progesterone, estradiol, cortisol, and vitamin D. Only a qualified physician or company that specializes in hormone optimization should interpret these results. Don't ever take this tool into your own hands. Be leery of all the antiaging advertisements out there on the Internet. Any antiaging claims that sound too good to be true usually are. Read the literature and educate yourself on hormone optimization first.

There are many age-management companies out there. You've probably seen the advertisements for Cenegenics Medical Institute with the seventy-three-year-old doctor with six-pack abs. That's Dr. Life, and yes, his story is real. Consider reading his book, titled *The Life Plan*, which discusses his nutrition and exercise program along with his hormone optimization plan through Cenegenics. Learn about how he got such a "shredded" body at his age. It's truly amazing.

Start thinking about all of your lifestyle behaviors. How important is it to you that you age better? Sound nutrition, physical activity, and a calm mind are the key ingredients to aging gracefully. You can achieve this over the course of time. Be patient. There's no magical pill that instills proper nutrition and exercise. Therefore, plan on shifting your energies toward maximizing the quality of your life for the rest of your life. You've gotta really want it.

EXERCISES

(1) Have I ever had my hormone levels checked?

(2) When do I plan on checking these levels and where?

(3) What are the top three symptoms I suffer from that may be due to poor hormone levels?

TOOL 52. PARK AT THE END OF THE PARKING LOT

If you're going to drive, you might as well park your car away from the entrance of wherever you're going. This increases your movement each day. I number this as a separate tool because it's that important. Parking far from building entrances also spares you from those careless individuals who push shopping carts or slam car doors into your car. Parking far away is a pain in the rear for most people, but the more movement you get in your day, the leaner you'll be. You aren't subtracting movement as you add exercise. You are adding more movement into your day with every opportunity *as well as* exercising, too.

Parking further away also adds steps to your pedometer. Let's have fun with this. If you park twenty spots away from a store entrance and each parking spot is approximately eight feet wide, multiply twenty by eight and you get an additional 160 feet of walking that day. Do this five days a week, and you'll add on an additional eight hundred feet of movement that week. Multiply this by four weeks and you'll walk 3,200 extra feet, which is 38,400 extra feet a year. Can you believe that parking you car away from the entrance equates to walking an extra 7.27 miles a year? Imagine you did this a couple of times a day? You can double the mileage each year. Ooh, now we're talking.

EXERCISES

(1) How many times did I park away from an entrance today?

(2) What did I do to take more steps today?

(3) Do I own a pedometer yet? (If *not*, buy a pedometer.)

TOOL 53. CLIMB A STEEP HILL EVERY WEEK

We tend to climb metaphoric mountains in our minds, whether it's at work or in our personal lives. These climbs can sometimes be challenging and prevent people from making an attempt.   Life consists of many intermittent steep hills. Going through a weight loss program is just another steep hill. It's time to unclutter your thoughts about this experience by transforming that mental climb into a physical climb so that you can reap the benefits of your accomplishment. Physically climbing a steep hill each week can help you embody a winning feeling after a mentally grueling day. The question is, how much power do you possess to conquer that hill? Will you stay at the foot of the hill and contemplate movement, or will you initiate the climb with the intention of finishing?

I love visualizing this exercise in my Spin classes. I take the students up several hills within the hour. When you climb a hill, you experience resistance that is physically and mentally demanding until you reach the top. Each time you succeed, it only reinforces a stronger confidence in your ability to be unstoppable. You must transfer that feeling of success to anything that's challenging for you in your life. It's all about keeping your level of commitment high and possessing that unstoppable mindset. You can also embody a steep hill by walking up a steep incline on the treadmill. As you conquer whatever hill you take on, in Spin class or on the treadmill, tell yourself that you can conquer anything in life. Never quit.

It's time to learn how to embrace life's challenges. How do these challenges help you get stronger? The same way climbing a physical hill does. You develop the muscle strength and endurance when you finish your climb. In life, you develop the mental and emotional strength when you conquer life's hills. Sometimes you may need help. Learn how to accept that help when it's needed.

This is why I love sports so much. Think of your favorite sports team. Each athlete faces different challenges from their opponents which require him or her to strategize every second of the game. To win, athletes must possess perseverance and trust in their teammates so that they can climb the toughest mountains against their most challenging opponent. Athletes train hard and learn to possess mental stamina to win the game. They study the opponent's style and tactics so as to use the right strategies to win. Athletes play to win. There is no *try* and no excuses holding them back from being their best.

Picture yourself as an athlete. Maybe you were an athlete growing up. Maybe not. Either way, let's ignite a winning desire in your heart to succeed during your transformation. Write down the top three barriers holding you back from having the fire you need. Do this every day. Now identify the tools you'll need to get through these barriers and then use them.

When I say climb a steep hill every week, I mean it. When you're done with the climb, your body is flooded with endorphins and other happy hormones. Climb whenever you can. Climb the stairs instead of taking the elevator. Physical fitness improves mental acuity and energy levels. By the time you get to your floor, you'll be ready to conquer any task with a clearer mind.

EXERCISES

(1) Is there a steep hill I can walk up near my neighborhood?

(2) What are the top three tools I need to successfully climb up this steep hill?

(3) How will bringing out the athlete in me help me through my weight-loss journey?

TOOL 54. JOIN A LEAGUE

A patient of mine hated exercise and was bored in the gym. I almost pulled out my tiny violin to play a sympathy song for him. Instead, I suggested that he join a sports league. Two years later, he is in the same basketball league and loves it. He gets to practice three days a week for a couple of hours each day, which provides him with plenty of cardiovascular exercise for the week. This is a great beginning. He has also hired a personal trainer he loves, which gets him through his weight-training program.

There are many leagues out there: bowling, softball, flag football, basketball, kickball, racquetball, squash, tennis, volleyball, crew, running, golf, and so many more. If you're not motivated to exercise in the gym, a league may be the way to go for you. Not only will it conjure up a competitive edge in you, but it will also give you a sense of belonging. A league allows you to meet new people, network, and get back into the groove of moving more.

My beautiful sister wanted to get back into great shape last year and wanted more than just the gym. She got involved in a Zumbathon, which was a dance recital. This gave her a sense of belonging with her Zistas (Zumba + sisters = Zistas), all of whom spent several weeks engaged in vigorous dance rehearsals. My sister got into amazing shape. To this day, she socializes with the Zistas and her body is out of this world.

Ask a friend to join a league with you. You'll feel so amazing deep down inside when you tell one of your colleagues, "I've got a softball game tonight. Wish us luck." People always respect adults who play sports in their thirties, forties, and even fifties. Just make sure that you stretch before playing, and choose a sport that you enjoy. Never overdo it, but always play to win. If you can put your best foot forward and be part of a winning team, you'll inherit a new outlook during your re-acclimation to fitness. Let's win a healthy way of life.

EXERCISES

(1) Which sport do I like to play?

(2) What is the closest public park to me, and which leagues do they offer?

(3) Whom will I invite to join the league with me?

TOOL 55. GET THE RIGHT SHOES

Get the right shoes for all day, every day, not just for your workouts. Healthy feet allow you to move more every day. I know you are probably more concerned about fashion than about personal comfort, but there are shoes out there that are cute and comfortable if you look for them.

Women, hear me out on this one because I may be speaking directly to you. Four-inch stiletto heels are not the right shoes. When your feet are put into high heels, your toes are pushed downward into what's called plantar flexion, which puts a large strain on the muscles in your foot, Achilles tendons, calves, and knees. In addition, chronic calf tightness can lead to a condition called plantar fasciitis, in which the sole of your foot is inflamed. This disorder sucks and can be easily avoided.

Consider getting wedges. They are fashionable and far more functional than any stiletto heel. Tight shoes that push your toes into a tight space like sardines in a can will also cause you major orthopedic problems later. You may always be tight and, on some level, in pain. Do you need another excuse not to exercise? No way! Just think—if all movement in the human body starts at the foot and affects the whole kinetic chain, then you must keep your feet healthy and free from any obstructions when walking. Incommodious shoes will cause you to overwork your ankles, knees, hips, spine, and neck.

Men, this tool applies to you, too. If you wear uncomfortable dress shoes or work boots, you'll suffer from the same types of problems. Therefore, consider comfortable shoes for work to decrease the risk of any injuries. It's bad enough that most people sit for a majority of their day. A combination of movement in the wrong shoes and the lack of movement from a sedentary job can eventually lead to an injury.

When it comes to working out, choose the right shoes, too. Runners should have two pairs of sneakers, a separate pair for running and your day-to-day sneakers. For movements that require a lot of side-to-side movement, consider getting a cross-trainer sneaker. Spinning students should get cycling shoes. Ask a qualified fitness expert or podiatrist in your area to check out your biomechanics (the way you move) and make suggestions for the right type of shoes for you.

EXERCISES

(1) What type of shoes do I wear on an average day?

(2) Do my feet hurt at the end of the day?

(3) How is my overall posture?

(4) Do I stretch my calves, hamstrings, and hips each day?

TOOL 56. CHECK LABELS

Do you know what you're putting into your mouth? Do you know how to read a food label? Let's keep this simple. I know it can be such a challenge to understand labels. Let's break it down using the label from a familiar food—oatmeal.

Nutrition Facts For Oatmeal

Amount Per Serving:	½ cup uncooked
Calories	150.0
Fat	2.5 g

Saturated Fat	0.0 g
Polyunsaturated Fat	1.0 g
Monounsaturated Fat	1.0 g
Cholesterol	0.0 mg
Sodium	0.0 mg
Potassium	0.0 mg
Carbohydrate	27.0 g
Sugars	1.0 g
Fiber	4.0 g
Protein	6.0 g

Vitamin A 0 %   Vitamin C 0 %

Calcium	2 %	Iron	10 %
Vitamin D	0 %	Vitamin E	0 %
Thiamin	0 %	Riboflavin	0 %
Niacin	0 %	Vitamin B12	0 %
Vitamin B6	0 %	Manganese	0 %
Phosphorus	0 %	Copper	0 %
Selenium	0 %	Magnesium	0 %
		Zinc	0 %

This oatmeal container lists a serving size of one-half cup uncooked oats. Most food labels base their nutrition facts on one serving, but others base it on two servings and sometimes more. You must measure out one serving and stick to it. Measure it accurately with a cup. Portion control is essential for weight loss.

Fat content is important to look at. There are saturated fats, polyunsaturated fats, and monounsaturated fats broken down under this category.

Saturated fat might lead to heart disease when eaten in excess. Avoid products that contain more than 10 percent saturated fat out of the total fat content.

Polyunsaturated fat contain omega 3s, which in the human body break down more easily and offer immediate bioavailability. Omega 3s can lower inflammation and decrease your risk of heart disease and certain cancers. You can consume your omega 3s from many sources including seeds, nuts, fish, algae, leafy greens, and krill.

Monounsaturated fat can protect your heart and decrease your risk of certain cancers. You can get monounsaturated fat from oils such as olive oil, peanut oil, and avocado oil. Other natural foods include high-fat fruits such as avocados and olives.

Cholesterol is listed on the oatmeal label as having zero mg. The label also states it's a cholesterol-free food. Make sure these claims meet set government standards. A cholesterol-free food must have less than two milligrams (mg) of cholesterol and two grams (g) or less of saturated fat.

Always look at the amount of added sodium in food. If you have high blood pressure (hypertension), you shouldn't exceed 1,500 milligrams of sodium each day. Anything above that can increase your blood pressure. If you don't have hypertension, you can eat as much as 2,300 milligrams of added sodium a day. Believe it or not, when you dine out, one meal may exceed these values. That's why the most common drugs for the brain are sugar and salt. We've been drowning our minds in this stuff, and when the high goes low, our brains shout, "Give me more!" Most nutrition experts will ask you to eat at home so that you can control how your food is prepared and eat the right serving size.

As you can see, oatmeal has twenty-seven grams of carbohydrates, four grams of which come from fiber. Fiber (tool 63) is necessary to keep your gastrointestinal health strong and your blood sugar in check. You should consume at least twenty-five grams of fiber a day.

Caloric intake should be commensurate with your RMR (tool 49). One serving of this oatmeal contains 150 calories. Choose food with the least amount of added sugar in it. Sugar causes insulin spikes, and we know that chronic insulin spikes cause you to be fat. My rule of thumb is that when you can, stick to less than ten grams of added sugar in one serving, and you're good to go.

The protein in oatmeal is six grams and comes from plants. Remember to get enough protein in each meal. Have you ever tried adding four cooked egg whites to your oatmeal? Super yummy!

Finally, I should mention that all labels list the micronutrient content in one serving, too. Micronutrients include all the minerals your body needs. They act as your spark plugs for chemical processes to occur in the body. Many people choose to supplement with a multivitamin since food doesn't contain optimal levels of micronutrients. Other popular supplements include fish oil, CoQ-10, magnesium, probiotics for the gut, calcium, and vitamin D. Ask your physician which supplements you should take. The quality of supplements depends on the brand.

Label reading is crucial. Now that you have an idea of what you're looking at, start looking at food labels with everything you eat.

EXERCISES

(1) When I rummage through my pantry, do I know which items belong based on what I've learned so far?

(2) How much added sugar did I consume today? How many total calories did I consume? How much protein did I consume?

(3) Which supplements do I need?

TOOL 57. DITCH THE SUGAR

Limiting your sugar intake will help you lose weight. Consuming too much sugar will have the following effects:

- Your blood sugar will go through the roof, and your insulin will chase right after it. This will cause you to hold onto fat and accumulate more fat over time.

- You'll always have severe sugar cravings.

- You'll experience glycation, which happens when proteins cross-link to sugars and form disruptive structures in the body that then disable proteins from doing their job. Remember, proteins are found in the skin, organs, and vascular structures, providing cohesion and elasticity for these systems. Proteins also form the enzymes in your body. Proteins help to build the immune system through antibodies, help with muscle contractions, are transporters that move molecules through the body, act as messengers for hormones, and store as amino acids for future use. In the end, glycation disrupts normal metabolic pathways and promotes diseases such as metabolic syndrome, cancer, diabetes, arthrosclerosis, and stroke.

- You'll age very quickly.

Do you want this to happen to *you*? I didn't think so. If this doesn't motivate you to reduce your sugar intake, then what will? Just because it's habit to grab a candy bar or big bowl of fruit in the afternoon doesn't mean you can't modify these behaviors today for a disease-free life tomorrow.

Don't be fooled by "low-fat" labels at coffee establishments and elsewhere. These items are *loaded* with sugar. When companies take out the fat, they curse you with added sugar and other junk ingredients so that you have something exciting to bite into.

Sugar is also found in juice. Juice bars contain sugar-loaded drinks, so avoid these places. Most people drink natural juices thinking that the sugar isn't high. This is not the case. All juices, no matter where they come from, have a lot sugar in them. Natural orange juice will always give you more than one serving of fruit per glass. Imagine drinking what may be equivalent to eight oranges in one large glass of orange juice! Not good! Remember to consume at most three servings of fruit a day. It's best to consume whole fruit compared to fruit juice. Stick to one serving of fresh-squeezed juice, which is under a cup, unless you exercise at a high intensity.

Eliminate high-glycemic carbohydrates, too (tool 68). These items include bread, pasta, rice, sweets, and potatoes. High-glycemic carbohydrates elevate blood-sugar levels quickly, which elicits the insulin response. I keep bringing up the perils of insulin release in the body because, as you know, large levels of insulin at any given time will debilitate your ability to burn fat. Although there is a big hype on whole grains, stay clear of high volumes of that stuff because you want your body to burn fat for fuel and not store it.

Some people ask me how often they can eat these foods. It's a loaded question because there's a place for everything. Theoretically, if your number-one goal is to decrease cravings and lose body fat, then I say get rid of them. Our bodies don't *need* these things to survive. We can survive without them since there are plenty of healthy alternatives available to us. We eat these things out of habit. So the rule of thumb is this: if you look at the label under carbohydrates and there's a listing for sugar, make sure the sugar is less than ten grams. Snack on food with natural sugars in it, such as carrot sticks, celery sticks, apples, peaches, pears, cherries, or grapes. You can even mix any of these with a fistful of nuts or dip your veggies in hummus. It's always wise to eat a carbohydrate (grains, veggies, and fruits) with a protein or healthy fat. For example, eat a pear with a fistful of almonds or a cup of berries with a cup of low-fat cottage cheese.

You can reverse the years of poor eating by adopting healthier eating patterns. Ask your doctor to run lab tests that include glucose, insulin, and hemoglobin A1c levels. These labs screen for diabetes. By knowing your numbers, you can see where your levels fall around the reference range. Ask your doctor if he or she is concerned about your results. Ditch the sugar and you'll turn your body into a lean machine.

EXERCISES

(1) What high-sugar foods do I currently eat?

(2) What can I eat instead?

(3) What are my glucose, insulin, and hemoglobin A1c levels?

TOOL 58. DRINK WATER

There are flavored waters, sugary waters, and waters sweetened with fake sugar. How about just plain old water?

Boring, I hear. Well, as a society, we've cut down on the amount of water we consume, and many people have increased their intake of diet sodas (yuck—aspartame), fruity juices (and no, these don't count as your daily fruit allowance), sweetened waters, lattes, power drinks, mineral drinks, age-defying drinks, drinks that are filled with potent antioxidants, drinks that calm you down, drinks that make you smarter—you name it. There are so many gimmicks out there and so many people buy into them instead of just drinking plain ol' water. Water always wins and it's actually a natural fat burner.

You should drink half your body weight in ounces a day. Add on another eight ounces for every hour of exercise you do and on hot days. So if you weigh two hundred pounds, you need one hundred ounces of water a day. That equals a little more than six standard sized water bottles a day. Drink water throughout the day to attain this. It seems like a lot, but water is the conduit for every physiological process in your body. Ample levels of fluid allow your cells to do their job. When you fail to drink enough water *and* you eat poorly, your cells become sticky and dehydrated. Your blood becomes thick, viscous, and dark. Your urine is bright yellow and dense rather than clear in color if you aren't well hydrated. Can you imagine how your poor kidneys feel? They're trying to push out excretion yet lack the proper medium, water, to transport the waste out. This can be detrimental to the gastrointestinal tract causing GI problems such as constipation.

The following are symptoms of water deficiency:

- Chronic fatigue
- Thirstiness

- Dry mouth, skin, and lips

- Hunger

- Headaches

- Muscle cramping

- General joint stiffness

Add optimal amounts of water into your day to help alleviate these symptoms. A well-hydrated body is a healthy body.

Don't drink your calories, especially during weight loss. To make plain water more interesting, you can always add fruit or cucumber slices. Ahh, refreshing.

EXERCISES

(1) How will I track my water intake each day?

(2) What do I currently drink too much of?

(3) Other than water, what will I drink each day?

TOOL 59. EAT PROTEIN BASED ON LEAN BODY WEIGHT

Not only should you eat small, frequent meals, but you should also consume enough protein throughout the day; otherwise, you'll overeat at night. By adding substantial amounts of lean, *organic* protein into your day, you'll end up eating fewer calories each day. This equates to more weight loss.

102.99

Eat one gram of protein per pound of lean body weight. This is not an industry standard. I personally found that this works well for my clients. I've told people to distribute this number of protein over five meals a day. This is just a starting point. Each individual has unique needs. You should be hungry every three to four hours. If you are too full to eat in that time block, then you need to decrease your protein by an ounce each meal. If you are hungry an hour or two after a meal, then increase your protein by an ounce. This is a dynamic process and depends on how active you are each day.

First, identify what your lean body weight is. When you get on a scale, you're weighing the total package. So if you have a big brain, then there's your answer. Just kidding. In all seriousness, focus less on the scale and more on what your body-fat percentage is. I know I keep mentioning weight loss throughout this book, but please know that I really mean fat loss. Revisit tool 50 to determine what your lean body weight is from your body composition measurement. Protein feeds that lean weight.

When I worked at a medical weight loss clinic, patients were always discouraged when the scale didn't reflect any weight loss. I spent a lot of time getting them to understand that people don't necessarily lose weight every day, and that weight loss encompasses fat loss and muscle gain. Remember, the more muscle you have, the higher your RMR (tool 49). As long as you're eating well and exercising, the weight will come off. It may take longer than you'd like but the goal is to create healthy lifestyle habits that reduce body fat, not just weight. Under severe caloric restriction, muscle is catabolized. By eating small, frequent meals that contain protein, low-glycemic carbs, and healthy fats, you may only lose ten pounds in a couple of months, but those ten pounds will come from fat versus muscle.

First, understand what a portion is. For example, if you need twenty-five grams of protein per meal, then that would equal approximately six large egg whites, four ounces of chicken, three-quarters of a cup of low-fat cottage cheese, or four ounces of salmon. Buy a kitchen scale and measure your food. Otherwise, *guestimate* the portion by using the size and thickness of your palm, not counting the fingers.

Once you find out how many grams of protein you need, you can figure out how many ounces you need of each protein source per meal. These are approximate values:

- Chicken breast: 6.6 grams/oz.

- Turkey breast: 6.1 grams/oz.

- Wild game: 8 grams/oz.

- Egg whites: 14.75 grams/half of cup

- Low-fat cottage cheese: 15 grams/half of cup

- Nonfat plain Greek yogurt (Fage, Voskos, or Chobani): 14 grams/6 oz.

- Mahimahi: 8.5 grams/oz.

- Salmon (wild): 6.1 grams/oz.

- Tuna (canned): 7.2 grams/oz.

- Tuna (fresh): 6.6 grams/oz.

- Whitefish: 5 grams/oz

- Shellfish: 4.8 grams/oz.

- Alternative sources: hemp protein, sprouted brown rice protein, pea protein (values vary)

- Vegan sources:

  o Tempeh: 15 grams/half of cup

  o Non-GMO tofu: 2 grams/oz

  o Nuts: 6 grams/24 nuts

  o Beans: 20 grams/half of cup

Protein feeds your muscle. Muscle is like a furnace. The more muscle you have, the more calories you'll burn each day.

EXERCISES

(1) Do I know which foods are considered protein?

(2) How many grams of protein do I need each day? For each meal?

(3) Do I own a kitchen scale? (Buy a cheap and reliable one from Bed, Bath & Beyond along with fun, colorful cups to measure fruits, vegetables, and other items.)

TOOL 60. EAT FIVE VEGETABLES AND TWO FRUITS A DAY

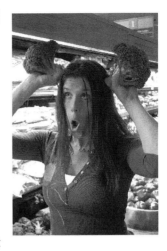

You realize that fruits and vegetables are considered carbohydrates, right? I ask you this because many people I work with state, "JZ has me eating no carbs." This isn't true. I get people off the high-glycemic carbs since it makes them bloated all the time. High-glycemic carbs also feed the sugar addiction. Mother Nature's best ingredients don't tend to bloat you and are vital to the body.

We need our fruits and veggies, which most people don't get enough of each day. For example, if lunch usually consists of a sandwich, then you're losing out on an opportunity to eat vegetables with that meal unless your sandwich contains a whole cup of vegetables on it. Getting five vegetables and two fruits in each day is the biggest challenge for most people. That is why sandwiches are not a good "staple" food. When you eat a sandwich, you skip the veggies.

Consider juicing your veggies in a blender. My favorite green drink consists of two cups of kale, two persian cucumbers, one granny smith apple, four large carrots, water and one ounce of ginger. Cut up all your veggies and fruits at the beginning of each week and place them into separate containers in your fridge. These foods are truly your best friends for weight loss and for life.

People tell me they eat so much salad, but when I see their portions, they still fall short of the daily recommendation of vegetables. Familiarize yourself with what a true portion is. For example, one whole cucumber or whole bell pepper equals one vegetable serving. Other examples include two cups of torn lettuce, kale, or spinach, one cup of asparagus, broccoli, brussels sprouts, celery, carrots, mushrooms, or onions. One fruit serving may include one small Washington apple, one citrus fruit, one pear, one peach, one plum, one apricot, or a half cup of berries. Avoid too many tropical fruits since they're higher in sugar.

Vegetables and fruits are loaded with antioxidants, nutrients, fiber, and vitamins. These natural foods help fight against diseases. So why do people skip them? Perhaps childhood aversions are to blame. Do you not have access to good-tasting veggies and fruits? Then grow them yourself. What a treat for you *and* your family. A garden is a picturesque scene in your backyard. There is something very special about eating your own crop. You grew it. You'll find it more enjoyable because the work has paid off once it's in your mouth. Garden-picked veggies and fruits on your kitchen counter will also stimulate your visual receptors so you want to eat them. Sweet!

Last, presentation is everything. Have you ever been to a catered event where the fruit platter is shaped like a paradise cove with dolphins made out of bananas and pineapple slices acting as blossoming flowers? How about a vegetable dish that is neatly cut up with cucumbers, fresh cherry tomatoes, celery sticks, cauliflower, broccoli, and zucchini surrounding hummus or a healthy dip? So yummy! Be creative with your veggies and fruits, and you'll notice you and your family want to eat them.

EXERCISES

(1) What creative way can I make fruits and vegetables more enticing for my family to eat?

(2) How many veggies and fruits do I currently eat? (I pledge to track this and master it.)

(3) How will I integrate more veggies into my daily nutritional plan?

TOOL 61. DITCH THE SODA

Soda is the worst ingredient for weight loss. I've worked with people who cut out soda and immediately saw and felt changes in their body. Your body will easily overcome this habit once you quit.

Most people drink diet soda thinking that it's better for them. The fact is, while regular sodas are loaded with sugar, diet sodas are loaded with chemicals such as aspartame and phosphoric acid. These ingredients can harm your body in the long run both neurologically and physically.

1) Aspartame is a potent neurotoxin, which can affect your endocrine system and nervous system by

bringing on the early onset of alzheimers and other neurological deficiencies.

2) Phosphoric acid can eat away at your bones by causing calcium loss.

3) Regular soda contains high-fructose corn syrup (industrialized sugar) which can cause poor development of collagen, copper deficiencies, liver problems, and possibly diabetes.

You can substitute soda with carbonated beverages such as Pellegrino or Perrier. Have you considered adding flavor to your water with a dash of lemon or berries? There are some sodas that use Stevia sweetener without the other harmful ingredients. However, I am a bigger fan of just plain ol' water and herbal tea. Sorry!

EXERCISES

(1) How many sodas do I currently drink a day?

(2) What beverage(s) will replace my soda habit?

TOOL 62. TAKE FISH OIL

When people diet they tend to decrease their fat intake. While some fats are not good for you, others are essential for weight loss and maintaining a healthy body. Fish oil

contains omega 3s, which help you produce the polyunsaturated fats that your body can't produce on its own.
Fats that your body needs but can't produce are called
essential fatty acids (EFAs) and can be obtained from food
and supplementation. You can get your EFAs from foods
containing omega 3s such as tuna, anchovies, seeds, nuts,
and wild Alaskan salmon.

Fish oil is an excellent addition to this list. Fish oil has wonderful anti-inflammatory properties, and when you have
chronic inflammation, weight loss can become a challenge.
There are many systems in the human body all running in
synergy with one another, and one system being off will
cause the others to suffer. When you combine healthy eating habits with regular exercise, you cut back on systemic
inflammation, which allows your body to operate much
more functionally.

Taking fish oil can help promote weight loss. This is what
happens: The omega 3 fatty acids from fish oil trigger fat-
burning enzymes in the body. Both exercise and omega 3
fatty acids increase your overall metabolic rate, which stops
pre-fat cells from storing as fat in your body. This process
allows your body to burn fat as fuel, which in turn will stimulate weight loss. Now that is what I call teamwork.

The quality of fish oil capsules differs from company to company. It's crucial to find a fish oil brand that has both DHA
and EPA in it. For some people, not having an aftertaste
is the most important factor when choosing their fish oil.
Others consider the size and the flavor of the capsule when
making their choice. Sometimes it takes trial and error to
find a fish oil that works best for you. Take two to four capsules of fish oil each day to decrease inflammation, aid in

stronger heart health, and to improve your cognitive function. Krill oil is also an excellent supplement, especially for people who can't take fish oil. Always consult your doctor before using any supplementation.

EXERCISES

(1) Which foods do I already eat that provide me with omega 3s?

(2) How much fish oil is good for me?

(3) What foods can I add into my nutritional plan that are rich in omega 3s?

TOOL 63. GET THAT FIBER

Very few people consume enough fiber each day. You need at least twenty-five grams of fiber. Fiber is a superstar in the body.

- It helps keep your gastrointestinal track clean. Think of fiber as a broom that sweeps the carcinogens out of your pipes so that all the disease-causing debris is pushed out of your body.

- It helps regulate blood sugars.

- It increases satiety (fullness).

Eat fibrous foods each day instead of foods that contain high-glycemic, refined carbohydrates and practically no fiber. Below are examples of high-fiber foods with proper portions and the approximate fiber amount per serving. Stick to the listed serving. Remember to distribute these foods throughout your day and eat them with a protein or healthy fat. Don't double your fruit portions to increase your fiber intake. If you do that, you'll end up eating too much sugar in one serving.

- 3 dried figs = 10.5 grams
- 2 dried apricots = 1.7 gram
- ½ cup raspberries = 4.6 grams
- ½ cup blueberries = 3.8 grams
- 1 cup strawberries = 4.4 grams
- 1 small apple = 4 grams
- 1 medium pear = 4 grams
- 1 large kiwi = 3.1 grams
- ½ granadilla passion fruit = 6 grams
- 1 small orange = 2.4 grams
- 1 small papaya = 2 grams
- 1 small mango = 4.5 grams
- ½ medium avocado = 12 grams
- ½ cup unsweetened coconut = 5 grams
- 1 cup cooked oatmeal = 6 grams

- 1 fistful sunflower seeds = 3.4 grams

- 3 Tbsp flaxseeds = 6.9 grams

- 1 fistful nuts (almonds, pecans, pistachios) = 3 grams

- ½ cup lentils = 6.8 grams

- ½ cup black beans = 7 grams

- 1 cup brussels sprouts = 3.6 grams

- 1 cup green beans = 4 grams

- 1 cup cooked carrots = 5.2 grams

- 1 small cooked sweet potato = 4.9 grams

- 1 cup turnip greens = 5 grams

- 1 cup cooked spinach = 4.3 grams

- 1 cup cooked peas = 8.8 grams

- 1 cup cooked zucchini = 2.6 grams

- 1 cup cooked kale = 7.2 grams

- 1 cup cooked broccoli = 4.5 grams

- ¼ cup quinoa seeds = 6.2 grams

- 1 cup cooked cauliflower = 3.4 grams

- 1 cup cabbage = 4.2 grams

- 1 small tomato = 1 gram

EXERCISES

(1) If I had to guess, how much fiber do I eat daily?

(2) Which items on this list will I incorporate immediately? (Highlight them.)

(3) What meal can I create using these foods? (Write it out and add a protein and/or healthy fat to it.)

TOOL 64. COOK AT HOME

When you eat out all the time, you are probably overeating calories, fat, sodium, and definitely carbohydrates. You also don't receive the best quality or preparation of meat vegetables, or whatever you're eating. I can't make this general statement for every restaurant establishment, but I will say that people tend to lose more weight when they eat food that was prepared at home.

Do you have any clue how restaurants prepare their food? Do you ever truly know how many ounces of steak you're eating when you eat out? Of course you don't. You shouldn't be eating more than four ounces of steak at any given meal, but most restaurants serve you a whopping eight to twelve ounce steak—easily. The same holds true for chicken, fish, and all other proteins—stick to the right portion (tool 59) for you. Most restaurants pride themselves on giving you a great value for the price they charge. In the toughest of economic times, people want value. I get that. If this is the case, then split the meal with whomever you're with. Otherwise, take home half so that you can eat the rest for another meal. Voila—you saved money!

It's important to fuel your body with the best quality food. When you prepare your own meal at home, you're in control of your portion size (using a kitchen scale and measuring cups) and the quality of food.

Cooking at home also keeps your family close. You can all debrief, laugh, and be a close unit. You can't top this! Family love is better fuel for the body than anything else in the world. If they're not into healthy eating, then find creative ways to make eating healthy a delicious and fun experience for them. Consider hosting a food trivia game to help boost their education on the different food groups. Learning at the dinner table over a healthy meal that actually tastes good will teach your family that eating healthy isn't always boring.

I have a great example. When I first met my fiancé, Alan, he weighed 238 pounds and I weighed 160 pounds. For a five-foot, nine-inch frame, 160 pounds doesn't seem all that bad. But since I'm an athlete, being twenty-two pounds more than what I weigh today needed to change immediately. I used to run eight miles on the beach back then. After running, I felt pain in my knees and lower back from carrying extra weight around. I remember lying on my living room floor and icing my joints after every run. I told Alan that it was time to lose weight.

We began a three-month journey together as a team to get the weight off. We did it aggressively. We bonded over healthy dinners. There were always leftovers. He cooked meals such as barbeque chicken or shrimp skewers with onions, peppers, pineapple slices, and cherry tomatoes. He accompanied the skewers with a big green dinner salad. After three months, he lost twenty-eight pounds, and I dropped twenty-two pounds. We felt at home again!

Having a support system helps a lot. But you must each find your own urgency factor to make the necessary changes. In other words, you each need your own source of motivation to change your lifestyle habits right now. Urgency means now. Not tomorrow or next week—today! Once you find your urgency factor, all you need to do is keep your eyes on the prize and move forward in that direction. For me, having no pain was my prize. For Alan, it was me. Ha ha.

EXERCISES

(1) When was the last time I had a home-cooked meal?

(2) How will I implement this tool with my family?

(3) What is my urgency factor?

TOOL 65. THROW OUT THE JUNK FOOD

When you keep your kitchen stocked with healthy food, it's so much easier to make the right choices. Go to the grocery store today and stock your kitchen with the best food. If you have a cupboard full of artificial and refined foods, then do yourself a favor and dump it all in the garbage or donate it to charity. If something can live in a box for more than a couple of weeks, chances are there's a sea of preservatives in there, and maybe even the lovely demon we all call hydrogenated oil, too. These ingredients keep the product's shelf life high, which is the only reason why survival kits employ such foods; they can withstand any natural disaster. If these products can withstand natural disasters, then what makes us think our bodies can break this stuff down? None of us are the Incredible Hulk. There's only one Lou Ferrigno, and even he eats healthy food.

The human body can't break junk food down efficiently. You will *not* lose weight, and you'll age very quickly on a junk-food diet. Be clear about what's considered junk food. The body needs chemical-free foods that come from Mother Earth. Our bodies are organic, so our food needs to be organic, too. Shopping the perimeter of the supermarket results in a healthy wagon full of JZ approved items. Those items on the out-skirted aisles include your produce section, dairy, seafood department, and meat department.

Let's think about this. Your kitchen may be what's keeping you unhealthy. How many times have you heard of a recovering alcoholic going to a bar just to hang out? My point exactly. The bar environment conjures up old desires and cravings, making it very hard for that person to avoid a relapse. The same goes for you with food. You must clear your kitchen of *anything* that can derail you from your weight-loss journey. The sooner you do this, the sooner you'll be leaner. Go into your kitchen after you're done reading this tool and get rid of the following:

- Wheat products

- White flour products

- Chips and crackers

- Heavy sauces that contain more than five grams of saturated fat

- Boxed noodles-n-cheese

- Boxed brownie mix

- Ice cream

- High-sugar juices

- High-sugar cereals that contain more than ten grams of sugar per serving

- Anything else with a shelf life longer than a month

Just get rid of it. If you have to think about it twice, it's probably not good for you. If you don't want to throw it out, then keep it, pollute your body one more time, and never buy this junk food again. Does that work better for you?

Once you ditch the junk, purchase these staple items to keep in your home:

- Unsalted nuts, pumpkin seeds, or sunflower seeds

- Low-fat cottage cheese

175

- Fresh berries
- Other fruits such as apples, pears, peaches, or plums
- Green beans
- Hummus
- Carrot sticks
- Nonfat Greek plain yogurt
- Cucumbers
- Laughing Cow cheese light
- Lox (smoked salmon)
- Chicken breasts
- Tuna
- Sweet potatoes
- Turkey slices
- Celery sticks
- Container of egg whites
- Broccoli
- Kale
- Spinach

I can keep going, but as you can see, this is all fresh stuff. Your body will love you when you feed it with true love— Mother Nature.

EXERCISES

(1) Which foods must I part with? (Write a list.)

(2) After discarding these foods, how empty is my cupboard?

(3) What is my healthy grocery list?

TOOL 66. TAKE MELATONIN

Melatonin is a hormone that our brains produce naturally to help promote normal circadian rhythms during sleep. We naturally release melatonin into the bloodstream from the itty-bitty pineal gland located in the brain. This hormone is released when the sun sets. There's a decline in melatonin production as we get older, so most middle-aged people are advised to take melatonin supplementation. The goal is to drift off into a deep sleep so that you feel rested the next morning. Melatonin regulates sleep; it doesn't induce it.

Melatonin is an over-the-counter pill that is under-regulated by the FDA, so consult your doctor before taking it. Some people don't benefit from melatonin and should avoid it, especially if they suffer from depression. Children are not advised to take it either.

Melatonin can help with the following:

- Sleep
- Blood pressure
- Normalize cholesterol levels
- Heart health
- Decrease risk of stroke
- Protect against stress-induced illness
- Enhance sexual desire

For more tips about sleep, see tool 29. There are many possible reasons for a lack of restful nights. Making changes in your nighttime activities may be the answer for a quality night's rest.

EXERCISES

(1) How many hours of *good* sleep do I get each night?

(2) Am I getting enough sleep?

(3) How are my blood pressure and cholesterol values?

(4) Have I spoken to my doctor about melatonin supplementation?

(5) Have I decreased nighttime activities before bedtime?

TOOL 67. DRINK PROTEIN SHAKES

I will always tell you to eat whole foods first before I tell you to supplement your meals. However, most people I work with are too busy to pack whole foods each day, and so they skip meals as a result. Under these circumstances, you're better off drinking a balanced protein shake as a snack in between meals versus skipping a meal. There are many brands out there. The rule of thumb is to choose a shake with the least amount of processing. If you can't pronounce the ingredients in it, then you should probably avoid that supplement altogether.

There are protein powder brands available depending on your personal preference. Protein powders containing more than ten grams of sugar should be avoided. Quality protein powder will not only help build lean body mass but it will also boost glutathione levels in your cells. Very briefly, glutathione is a potent antioxidant that helps you fight against oxidative stress, viruses, and bacteria in the body. This type of protein is absorbed by the gut and is quickly distributed to your muscle cells for quick cellular repair after an awesome workout.

Some people like quick options that don't require a blender. In some cases, you can simply buy a shaker that blends powder and water. There are also some pre-made ready-to-go drinks that are sold in supplement shops, grocery stores, and online. Do not drink more than one of these a day. You don't want to risk overconsumption of heavy metals that may be in such drinks. Some people may even have sensitivities to some of the ingredients in protein shakes. Keeping a food journal (tool 28) allows you to identify if this is an issue for you.   You will want your trainer or nutritional coach to guide you in selecting the best brand for you.

As for any supplements, please note that protein supplements aren't regulated by the FDA. Be cautious that you don't consume too much protein in one sitting, including from protein supplementation. Purchase only reputable brands that don't contain lots of heavy metals or other chemicals. Learn to read labels (tool 56) and follow the serving size that best fits your recommended daily intake.

Make a social event out of taste testing protein shakes. Consider arranging a happy hour at your house one Friday night and try different protein shake recipes with close friends. Encourage your friends to compete in a contest to determine who can produce the best recipe. This will offer everyone good nutritional support while being in good company. Consider offering the person with the award winning recipe a canister of protein powder, a blender, or a gift card to Whole Foods or Trader Joes.

Here are a few of my favorite protein shake recipes:

Strawberry Shortcake
8 ounces water

5 frozen strawberries

¼ cup blueberries

2 tablespoons fat-free ricotta cheese

1 scoop vanilla protein powder

Chocolate Coffee Blizzard

8 ounces black iced coffee

1 scoop chocolate protein powder

½ cup shaved ice

Holiday Wonderland

8 ounces water

½ cup ice

Cinnamon to taste

Nutmeg to taste

1 tablespoon walnuts

½ teaspoon vanilla

1 scoop vanilla protein powder

JZ Especial

8 ounces water

½ cup ice

½ banana

1 scoop chocolate protein powder

1 tablespoon organic peanut butter

EXERCISES

(1) What meal am I most likely to skip and replace with a protein shake?

(2) When is my first happy hour?

(3) Which protein shake recipe won?

(4) What will be the prize for the contest?

TOOL 68. DITCH THE HIGH-GLYCEMIC CARBS

High-glycemic carbohydrates elevate your blood sugar and ultimately accumulate body fat, specifically in your trunk and belly region. Whenever you have repetitive sugar spikes throughout your day, you gain fat. I have met a lot of people who cut their portions down but don't reach their weight-loss goal due to high-glycemic carbohydrate consumption. This frustrates many people, and they eventually quit. Quitting is never the answer.

Reflecting on American history, with the rise of the obesity epidemic, we see that the Industrial Revolution is to blame. In time, diet gurus began to replace white-floured foods with whole-wheat items and claimed that there would be significant improvements in people's body composition. This isn't the case. Diseases such as diabetes and metabolic syndrome are more common now than ever before. Whole wheat is just as destructive to your weight-loss goal as white flour is. It may also be destructive to your overall health. Most people are shocked when I tell them to cut out all bread from their diet. Their first response is "Even wheat bread?" Yes, even wheat bread. Most people are sensitive to any refined high-glycemic carbohydrates. These types of carbs deter weight loss. You need carbs from veggies and fruits instead (tool 60). It's important to keep a daily food journal to identify what's working for you and what isn't. One tip that you should never forget; all carbohydrate consumption should be accompanied by a protein and/or healthy fat to avoid erratic blood sugar spikes. This will also lower the glycemic index for that meal.

Transitioning away from a high-glycemic to low-glycemic lifestyle requires you to first understand which foods are high glycemic and which ones are low glycemic. To keep it simple, high-glycemic carbohydrates include bread, pasta, rice, sweets, cereals, and potatoes. Cut out every high-glycemic carbohydrate for at least four-weeks. This will help you master the consumption of low-glycemic carbohydrates since these will be the only ones available to you. After four weeks, you'll realize that you don't even miss the high glycemic carbs. Your energy levels will be significantly higher, your weight will drop quicker and your waistline will get dramatically smaller.

Over-consumption of high-glycemic carbohydrates causes glycation (tool 57). Glycation is a word you'll hear a lot of in the future. Glycation disrupts normal metabolic pathways of all the cells in your body, which promotes the formation of diseases including heart disease, loss of hearing, metabolic syndrome, cancer, diabetes, atherosclerosis, and stroke. To prevent glycation from occurring, eat more low-glycemic carbs compared to high-glycemic carbs. You should especially avoid all high-glycemic carbs at night. Nighttime insulin spikes will make you fatter and also disrupt sleep, which causes sugar cravings the next day for an emotional and mental pick-me-up. Poor sleep patterns may alter your production of the two hormones responsible for maintaining energy balance; ghrelin (hunger) and leptin (fullness and appetite suppression). This imbalance will throw off your ability to stop eating and potentially causes more frequent hunger. Optimal physiology begins with the right nutrition.

Below is a list with portions of low-glycemic carbohydrates that you can consume without worrying about impeding weight-loss. Remember to eat all fruit in moderation. Please keep in mind that if it's green, you don't need to count the portion.

LOW-GLYCEMIC CARBS

Apple—1 medium
Apricot (dried)—half of cup
Artichokes*
Asparagus*
Bananas (under ripened)— half of small
Beans (virtually all beans)—half of cup
Blackberries—half of cup
Blueberries— half of cup
Broccoli*
Brussels sprouts*
Cabbage*
Carrots—1 cup
Cauliflower*
Cherries—1 cup

Cucumber*
Eggplant*
Garlic*
Ginger*
Grapefruit (ruby red)—half
Grapes—1 cup
Green beans—1 cup
Green peas—1 cup
Honey—2 tablespoons
Hummus—quarter of cup
Kale*
Lettuce*
Mango—1 medium
Mushrooms—1 cup
Onion*
Orange—1 small
Peach—1 medium
Pear—1 medium
Plum—1 medium
Raspberries—half of cup
Spinach*
Strawberries—1 cup
Sweet potato—half of cup
Tomato—1 medium
Yam—half of cup
Zucchini*
*However much you want

EXERCISES

(1) Do I own a measuring cup?

(2) If I had to guess, what percentage of my daily food intake consists of high-glycemic carbohydrate consumption?

(3) Which high-glycemic carbs can be easily eliminated from my nutrition?

(4) Out of the low-glycemic carbs, which are my top ten favorites?

TOOL 69. DRINK GREEN TEA EVERY DAY

Green tea is an ancient remedy with many health benefits. Through decades of usage, we know that green tea contains potent levels of antioxidants and nutrients that can potentially fight cancer and heart disease, lower cholesterol, aid in lipolysis (fat burning), stave off neurological deficiencies such as dementia, and remedy against diabetes and stroke. How come not everyone is drinking this stuff?

The antioxidants and other compounds found in green tea and other herbal teas help facilitate good health. As you may already know, antioxidants are nutrients that include vitamins, minerals, and enzymes that help your cells fight off the damaging effects of cellular oxidation. Oxidative stress occurs when the production of harmful molecules called free radicals damage both the protein and the genetic material, called DNA, in the cells. To create a visual of what oxidative stress looks like on the cells, picture an apple with a bite mark in it. Recall how that apple turns brown after allowing it to sit for an hour on a counter? That's what cellular oxidation looks like. Antioxidants aid in keeping cells healthy so that they don't brown like that apple. Antioxidants also boost your immune system and act as detoxifying agents that give you more energy.

Decaffeinated green tea and herbal tea are good replacements for late night snacking. The tea shifts your focus from food to a state of relaxation. Its warmth offers you comfort which was previously filled through late night snacking.

However, consuming caffeinated green tea before noon (tool 70) will help you burn fat because caffeine aids in thermogenesis. There are many green tea brands out there. Choose a natural green tea that doesn't have any added sugar in it. Sugar has calories. Stop drinking your calories.

EXERCISES

(1) After drinking green tea for a week, how are my energy levels and overall mood?

(2) Have I successfully eliminated my late night eating by drinking tea?

TOOL 70. ELIMINATE THE PM CAFFEINE

Limit your caffeine intake to the morning only. I know everyone has a different level of tolerance to caffeine, but most people who drink caffeine all day long experience low energy levels throughout the day and sleep poorly. Caffeine stimulates your mind and wakes you up. You won't need caffeine pick-me-ups when you eat the right food during the day.

Your early morning cup of joe doesn't need to change. But if you spend your entire day consuming coffee or diet soda (ugh!) then you're consuming way too much caffeine. Caffeine can disrupt your circadian rhythms and throw off your sleep patterns (tool 29).

Excessive amounts of caffeine also exacerbate anxiety and mood swings. I wouldn't want to be around that kind of person, would you? You don't have to be that person. Eat the right nutrition and you won't be. The more consistent you are with eating right, the more energy you'll have and the less you'll need caffeine.

Other consequences of excessive caffeine consumption include the following:

- Increased blood pressure

- Higher production of stomach acidity, leading to poor digestion

- Stomach irritation

- Interrupted digestion

- Potential dehydration (Remember; water is important for weight loss.)

- Increased incidences of osteoporosis in women, according to a report by the *American Medical Journal*

- Nervousness (which causes overeating)

- Irritability, agitation, headaches, or ringing in the ears (This can all lead to overeating due to frustration from the above symptoms.)

- The chronic release of cortisol in your bloodstream from your adrenal glands (Cortisol is the hormone associated with stress. Your body will hold onto body fat if cortisol is circulating at high levels due to stress.)

- Increased adrenal hormones, which increases blood sugar secretion, thereby stimulating the pancreas to produce insulin (Ooh, that insulin is back in the saddle again. Not good at all!)

Cutting back to one or two cups of coffee in the morning and ditching the caffeine after noon is a step in the right direction. Eating the right meal combinations will allow you to stick to this. This change will improve your energy levels throughout the day and calm your mood down. Eliminating the p.m. caffeine means eliminating all beverages containing caffeine such as espresso, cappuccino, and especially soda and diet soda, which you shouldn't be drinking anyway.

Avoid sweeteners in your coffee. A plain cup of joe in the morning is always best. You can even use skim milk or some cream.

EXERCISES

(1) How many caffeinated beverages do I drink a day?

(2) Which symptoms listed above do I experience?

(3) What is my plan of action for decreasing my caffeine consumption after noon?

TOOL 71. CREATE A NEW RECIPE

The formula for weight loss is to consume minimal sugar, eat natural foods, eat the right amount of each macronutrient (fats, protein, and carbs), drink plenty of water, sleep, have minimal stress, find love in your heart, and of course, exercise. When you mix these ingredients together, you get one amazing human being.

When it comes to choosing the right recipes for meals, have fun by creating new ones. Who says that healthy meals can't taste good? I love creating new recipes that are low in sugar but high in taste, and sharing them with neighbors and friends. I also share easy meal ideas on my blog www.JZfitness.com. Everyone should enjoy eating well. There's no need for healthy food to be boring. When people think of going on a diet, they think of being chained down to boring food. Dieters feel trapped and socially isolated. My question is always "Who makes you feel this way?" You do! You must dismiss these types of thoughts because they hold you back from change.

If I hadn't learned healthy ways of yummy eating, I would be so overweight. I am cursed with both a sweet tooth *and* a salty tooth. Double whammy for me! But I am lean because I eat *fun* healthy food. The key word is *fun*! I love eating yummy food just as much as you do. I'm an athlete, so my attitude is that I should be able to eat whatever I want. But my engine needs only the best fuel for optimal performance.

My engine can burn through a cookie, but its performance won't be as great. Suboptimal food makes me feel tired and stuffed like a pig every time. I can't stand that feeling. I therefore choose healthy foods. Learn how to modify restaurant menus, home-cooking recipes, and party menu planning. Here are some sample ideas:

- Instead of crackers and cheese, choose a whole cucumber sliced with a quarter cup of hummus.

- Instead of a bagel and cream cheese, choose once slice of Ezekiel bread toasted with one tablespoon of light Laughing Cow cheese, three ounces of lox, and two slices of heirloom tomato.

- Instead of meat lasagna, how about a turkey eggplant lasagna?

- Instead of pizza, how about a pizza with an almond-flour base crust, low-sugar sauce, two ounces of low-fat goat cheese, tomato, and fresh basil?

- Instead of chicken and rice, try lean turkey chili filled with veggies, such as peppers, onion, asparagus, and broccoli with sweet potatoes and no rice.

- Instead of a huge BBQ-and-ranch chicken salad, how about that same salad with all dressings on the side and nothing fried?

- Instead of an ice cream sundae, choose three-quarters of a cup of low-fat cottage cheese with chocolate-covered cashews and half a cup of blueberries.

It's always fun when you create a new recipe for the people you love. For example, one night I decided to substitute white flour with almond flour and made the best chocolate chip cookies ever for my colleagues. They were delicious and quite filling. Almond flour is higher in fiber, protein, and fat, which is why the cookies are satiating compared to regular sugary flour cookies. By no means will a cookie satisfy your day's need for fiber and protein, but it was amazing to me how delicious these gluten-free cookies were and how we can once in a while eat these types of things without feeling guilty about it. Now my office asks for these cookies all the time. Gosh, I may open up a healthy cookie bakery. Ha.

Another recipe I've mastered is my turkey gumbo. Instead of fattening chili, I mindlessly toss the following ingredients into a pot: a whole container of lean ground turkey meat, one minced red onion, garlic, three chopped peppers, two cups of broccoli, a little bit of sea salt, cayenne pepper, crushed red pepper, one cup of garbanzo beans, and two chopped up sweet potatoes. This gumbo makes approximately four meals.

Educate yourself on which ingredients are good for you. If it has added sugar, lots of sodium, high saturated fat, little fiber, low protein, and is high in calories, then avoid it. Trust me, a lean body doesn't benefit from any of this stuff. Lean people watch out for this stuff every day. In time, you'll be lean, too. Consider creating a cookbook with winning recipes that you and your friends invent, and then sell the book for charity. Make this journey fun.

EXERCISES

(1) How can I make a hamburger healthy? What should I serve with it?

(2) Can I think of a new chicken recipe?

(3) Design a dish for a vegan (tool 59 provides vegan protein sources).

(4) Which friends will I invite to create a healthy recipe cookbook with me?

TOOL 72. GET HOME-DELIVERY SERVICE

When there aren't enough hours in the day, treat yourself to your own personal chef or delivery service and give yourself a break, even if you only use the service for a couple of weeks at a time. Eating gourmet food that's correctly proportioned and healthy for you will help you achieve your weight-loss goal. It may be expensive; however, there's nothing more awesome than having your food prepared for you when time is tight and you can't cook. There are reasonable options out there when you search hard enough. You will always have my vote when it comes to investing in your health.

For example, I personally work with an excellent California-based company called Zen Foods (www.zenfoods.com). Their menu is extensive and delicious. The owners know my style of meal preparation, so just tell them to do it *JZ style* if you hire them. There are others out there if you look in your area.

Don't allow laziness and lack of time to prepare meals sidetrack you. Not only will delivery services create your food journal (tool 28) for you, but they package each meal individually, allowing you to consume the right amount of protein, carbs, and fat for each meal. Can you ask for more than that?

Delivery services also prove my point that healthy meals can taste like "real" food. I mean, come on, isn't that the biggest reason why you quit eating well in the past? You probably got bored eating bland food. If so, you never truly learned how to eat or cook yummy healthy food. Healthy food doesn't have to taste bland. It's actually quite tasty when a dash of love and effort are thrown into the meal preparation.

EXERCISES

(1) What are two local delivery services that I will call?

(2) After speaking with them, what did I like and dislike about each service?

(3) Who will I hire?

TOOL 73. STOCK YOUR KITCHEN WITH FOODS YOU DON'T CRAVE

My client once told me that she can't keep delicious food in her house because she'll eat it all in one sitting. That includes sweets, bread, ice cream, and cake. I told her, "You shouldn't eat this stuff anyway." However, this goes for everything. She once went shopping at the farmers market and purchased approximately eight pieces of fruit, all of which she ate that night. You're probably questioning why this is bad when fruit is good for you. It is, until it's eaten in such excessive amounts. Too much sugar. Anything in excess will be a physiological nightmare for your body. Another time she consumed almost a whole jar of organic peanut butter. While peanut butter contains healthy fat, eating a sixteen-ounce jar of peanut butter is 2,520 calories and 196 grams of fat, which is just awful! This one "meal" was double the calories she needed for the day. Sound familiar? Don't own any junk food. Peanut butter in this scenario is junk food. Junk food in your home creates an unsafe environment for you. Your home must breed healthy habits. Stock your fridge with the items listed under "Throw Out the Junk" in tool 65.

Your home is your work zone for self-improvement and change. Don't put yourself in an environment that isn't conducive to weight loss. Many people rationalize that the junk in their refrigerator is for their children and not for them. Well, that's even worse. Do you want your children to grow up to be obese or diabetic? If not, then you must start teaching them good healthy habits when they're young. You can only do this by adopting those habits yourself. Make sure you reward your family with outside treats such as chocolate, ice cream, or pizza once in a while so they don't feel completely isolated from the world. Consider scheduling *free days* twice a month, and enjoy ice cream sundaes as a family. When it's outside of the house, it won't be a staple food for your household. It will be an occasional treat.

I understand how much of a challenge this is. My staple food as a child was fast food. In my adult life, I had to reestablish a healthy foundation of what healthy eating was. If I can do it, so can you. Remember; take it one step at a time. Start by stocking your kitchen with healthy foods that you need to eat, rather than with the foods you love to eat. Breaking your chains means ending your love affair with food and learning to love your health more.

EXERCISES

(1) As I look through my pantry and refrigerator, which items need to go?

(2) Which items are hard to give up?

(3) What is my *new* staple grocery list?

TOOL 74. MODIFY THE MENU

Being on a weight-loss journey doesn't mean you can't eat out. There may be times when you join friends at a restaurant, celebrate a special occasion, or have a business dinner to attend. Don't be afraid to go. Simply learn how to modify restaurant menus so you can continue losing weight and feeling great.

A client of mine said that wherever she goes, there's never anything healthy for her to eat. I understand that chefs pride themselves on good taste, richness, and presentation. This means that sauces and lots of sugar are added to your dish. As good as the food may taste, your gut and body don't need it. It's perfectly okay to tell the server that you don't want any sauces or dressings anywhere on your meal. This includes salads and steamed veggies. Put it all on the side. If a meal contains bread, then substitute the bread with a sweet potato. The healthier the meal, the fewer the times your body will experience erratic insulin spikes.

So where do you start? When you're out with friends and they order poorly, you should order healthy even if it costs you a few extra bucks. Don't be scared of paying extra. For example, at breakfast, some restaurants charge extra for egg whites. Other restaurants charge you extra for modifying side dishes such as vegetables instead of french fries. The health benefits you gain from paying extra for healthy food is worth it. Ordering healthy in restaurants has become a trend. You wouldn't be the first person to ask the waiter to change how food is prepared. Be among the educated consumers and order healthy from now on. Don't be scared of being judged either. Your friends may laugh at you, but in the end when you're lean, they'll be begging you to reveal your secrets on how you did it.

I recently dined out at a prestigious restaurant in Beverly Hills and modified my meal even though I was out with a "very important" individual. The entrée was listed as steamed Virginia striped bass, Hong Kong style: garlic, chili oil, ginger, bok choy, baby carrots, shitake mushrooms, snap peas, jasmine rice, or brown rice. This was the exact listing on their menu. I asked the waiter, "Is there sauce on the sea bass? If so, can you kindly put that on the side? In addition, are the vegetables sautéed in a sauce? Can you put that sauce on the side as well? Last, can I sub extra grilled veggies instead of rice?" It's that simple. Don't care about what anyone says or does around you. The individual I dined out with actually ordered the same dish that I did since I sounded so "precise and health conscious."

Still not comfortable? Let's look at a couple of scenarios and my suggested solutions:

Scenario 1: You're at an event where they're serving salad loaded with dressing, bacon, and blue cheese. The main course includes ravioli; chicken parmesan with bacon, cheese, and breading; and a fatty-cut steak with mashed potatoes and fried onion rings on top. This recently happened to me—I'm not making this up.

Solution: Ask the waiter if they have a plain salad they can bring you with dressing on the side. Eat one piece of red meat the size of your palm without the mashed potatoes or fried onion rings. Eat two raviolis. This is more than enough food for you. Drink lots of water and grab a hot tea.

Scenario 2: Your whole family wants to eat refined carbs (pasta, bread, rice, potatoes, and sweets), but you're ready to eat low-glycemic carbs and don't want to cook two different meals.

Solution: Simply cook healthy meals for the entire family and don't even advertise it. Healthy dining is actually delicious when you do it right. For example, instead of spaghetti, try spaghetti squash with vegetables blended in. Add fish, chicken, or lamb in a low-sugar tomato sauce. They will love this dish.

Scenario 3: You're out to dinner for business, and everyone is ordering cocktails, sharing appetizers, and eating whatever they feel like eating. And then there's you, the one who's trying to lose weight.

Solution: As Dr. Joe Turcillo once told me, have quiet dignity. When everyone is passing around the plate, skip it and say, "No thank you!" Order a single glass of red wine, a protein (with no sauce) with a side of steamed veggies, and a sweet potato. Order a side salad as an appetizer with a light balsamic dressing on the side so you're eating something while everyone else is diving into the bad stuff. Who cares if you're not joining them? They don't have to go home after dinner feeling bad about messing up—you do. Be your own person in this situation and simply do what works for you. Who knows? Maybe others in your company will follow you. If they don't, it's not your problem.

EXERCISES

(1) How will I modify the menu from a restaurant that I plan on dining out at? (Go online and become familiar with their menu.)

(2) What will I do if people around me roll their eyes at how I order?

Chapter 4

MOTIVATION TO DO IT

You know what you need to do. The question is, will you do it? Everyone is impacted differently by different things. What motivates you may not motivate someone else. You must determine what motivates you. Don't think about tomorrow, and don't question why yesterday's motivation didn't work today. Be in the present; be in the now.

TOOL 75. SET UP TIME FRAMES FOR YOURSELF

Many people ask me how long it will take them to reach their goal. I sometimes want to reach into a hat and pull out an answer to that question. In other words, who knows? I know you don't want to hear this. You want a definitive answer. But everyone is different. If I had to guess, I would say that most people can lose one to two pounds most weeks *when they behave*. The rate at which you lose weight also depends on how much you need to lose. The weight will eventually slide right off ya when you consistently adopt healthy lifestyle behaviors. When I say *consistently*, I mean you are forever committed to the journey. Be patient.

Set up realistic time frames for yourself. For example, if you have more than twenty-five pounds to lose, then give yourself *at least* six months to do so. Six months is certainly enough time when you're *consistent*. You might feel that six months is too long to visualize. If this is true, then shorten the time frame to one-month increments. Set your goal up to lose four pounds a month. This may not impress you, but realistically you'll never be disappointed. If you lose more, then it's a bonus. Bonuses are always the best, aren't they?

Wanna be more aggressive? The larger the goal, the more work you must put in. This means committing five to six days a week every week to vigorous exercise, eating zero high glycemic carbs (tool 68), and paying attention to the fine details every day. Walking is not a form of vigorous exercise. Interval training is. Lifting weights is also part of the equation. Be specific with your time frames and be accountable to your goals. You can always be motivated and coached by me if you desire. Visit me at www.JZfitness.com.

Be specific with the goals you set for yourself. Determine how many times a week you'll exercise, the type of exercise you'll do, and the meals you'll consume.

Make your time line visual. Put your weekly goals up using a corkboard, chalkboard, dry-erase board, colorful poster boards, or whatever works for you. Pick a place to hang your time line. Be sure to position it in a place where you can see it every day. Make sure you stick to your time line by holding yourself accountable.

EXERCISES

(1) What do my time frames look like?

(2) How will I measure my success with each time frame?

(3) Which visual tools will I use on my time line to help me reach my goals?

TOOL 76. BE YOUR OWN BFF

When I was in high school, I had a BFF, which stood for "best friend forever." I remember how special I felt having that title. My BFF made me feel great, and I relied on her to get me through life's trials and tribulations growing up. It was always comfortable knowing that my BFF would always be there for me. But as we grew up, we grew apart. Different colleges split us up, and long-distance phone calls were expensive back then. As sad as this breakup was, I realized then that BFFs can be replaced.

I parallel this story to the BFF you find in food. As we learned earlier, there's definitely a link between finding comfort in the food (tool 15) we choose as our BFF. As comfortable as food makes you feel, it has kept you at an uncomfortable weight for all of these years. Therefore, it's time to break up with food and find a new BFF moving forward.

When we were children, food was often our reward. Remember when things went wrong or even went right, our parents or grandparents gave us lollypops, cookies, or other food that made us smile? Food instantly shifted our world away from rocky grounds to smooth, blossoming meadows. Our vulnerability was fed as children. We were instantaneously safe when we were handed a treat. As children, we bit into junk food knowing that everything was going to be okay.

As adults, we're desperate for that same comfort and safety. Most people feed their inner child to feel safe again. If you don't acknowledge this, it could decrease your ability to change your patterns of behavior. The only way to accomplish this is to be conscious every single day and find new tools to help break your chains from comfort food.

Choose to eat food to live, not to live to eat food. Choose to behave like a lean person if that's who you wish to be. Most lean people are go-getters. When life seems unbearable for lean people, they hit the gym, go for a hike, or do something that makes them feel mentally, emotionally, and physically great. Lean people don't play into feeling tired or unmotivated to work out. Lean people know that after their workout they feel like a million bucks. Lean people also use positive self-talk to help them feel good about themselves every day. The work it takes to do this always pays off when it's done. It's all about shifting your love away from food and into yourself by creating a healthy mind and body.

There are many ways of rewarding yourself after a hard day's work other than eating unhealthy food. First, figure out which tools will motivate you. Decide that you are no longer BFFs with food. You will no longer need food for comfort. *It's time to resolve unresolved issues.* The demise of your friendship with food will feel disheartening for a while. Find new outlets today. There are many tools in this book to help you succeed. Use them.

Do something healthy for your mind and body every day. Remember, being your own BFF can enhance your ability to sustain a healthy lifestyle.

EXERCISES

(1) What has been holding me back from being my own BFF?

(2) What's my first step to becoming my own BFF?

(3) What are the top three reasons why food is my worst BFF?

TOOL 77. LOOK AT PHOTOS

Past pictures of yourself help to remind you of how great life was when you lived in a leaner body. Start with a photo from when you weighed 10 percent less than what you weigh today. For example, if you're 200 pounds then find a picture of yourself at 180 pounds. What were you doing at 180 pounds? Start incorporating these behaviors into your life again.

Even though this may not be your final goal weight, it's a start. For some of you who have more than twenty-five pounds to lose, it can feel overwhelming. However, when you do it this way, it doesn't feel like a defeating journey. Even if you lose 10 percent, you'll be happier and actually healthier. Your photo should best represent who you want to be again. Put the photo where you can see it every day. Put it in your car, on your refrigerator, on your door, or in your planner. Visual aids are very powerful.

I remember a patient told me that he was most happy with his weight when he was younger. He ate fast food every day and never gained weight. Now that he's older and eating significantly better, he is unable to lose anything substantial. This is very frustrating for him. He told me that he was the high school football team star. His life embodied long practices that lasted for a minimum of three hours a day. Now, at the age of fifty-four, he may not be eating fast food, but he also doesn't exercise like he used to. Today, breads, crackers, and processed foods keep him overweight. Like him, people don't realize that eating poorly doesn't simply mean eating fast food. It also refers to consuming a diet that is rich in high glycemic carbohydrates (tool 68). For my patient, looking at his past photos reminded him of the vitality he once possessed, which motivates him today. Try this out for yourself!

EXERCISES

(1) What photo of myself from the past will inspire me today?

(2) What was my lifestyle back then?

(3) What life changes have I undergone since taking that photo?

TOOL 78. PURCHASE THE POUNDS

This is fun! Let's say you lost five pounds. Purchase a five-pound bag of whole-grain flour or place five pounds of canned goods in a grocery bag. Accumulate your weight so that you can *feel* your progress and for every twenty pounds you lose, donate the cans to charity. Visual and tactile tools are awesome motivators. I actually have a five pound fat replica in my office that I bought on Amazon which turns my patients off when they hold it. I calculate how many pounds of fat they have and tell them how many of those fat models they have in their bodies. Their demeanor instantly changes. Take note of what five pounds or ten pounds feel like, and realize that this was once part of your body. Five pounds is actually a big deal, and ten pounds, an even bigger deal. Reflect on every five pounds you lose.

I have a client whose goal is to lose twenty-six pounds. She has already lost thirteen and gained back three. In essence, she is still down ten pounds. I saw her losing focus. So before training her one day, I bought her ten pounds' worth of whole-grain flour wrapped in plastic placed in a gift bag. When she lifted the gift bag, she said, "Whoa, this is heavy! What's this for?" I told her that I was proud of her, and despite her gaining three pounds back, she was still doing well. She appreciated this gesture because her weight gain was due to a stressful job. She needed comfort food. This happens. I call it a hiccup in the road. Don't let that BFF (tool 76) try to get back into your life again. It caused you to be overweight in the past! Ditch the habit of regression, and keep lifting your pounds of success every time you fall away slightly. Catch your fall and find your balance.

If you have more than ten pounds to lose, this tool is priceless because the more you lose the more cans you'll donate to charity. Calculate how many hungry mouths you'll feed by dropping your weight. What a blessing in disguise.

EXERCISES

(1) Do I truly know how heavy ten pounds is?

(2) What were my thoughts as I lifted the pounds of progress?

(3) Which charity will I donate the food to once I hit my goal?

TOOL 79. BUY A POSTER OR PAINTING DEPICTING GOOD HEALTH

A picture of fruits, vegetables, or an image related to fitness will help you visualize a healthy and active lifestyle. These posters are your visual affirmations. I personally love affirmations. I have a lululemon poster that's full of healthy quotes. One of them is "Successful people replace the words *wish, should,* and *try* with 'I will!'" Isn't that a concept?

Redefine your overall experience with food. Little reminders strategically placed throughout your house and workspace will convince your subconscious mind to live in good health. Start by having a fruit bowl and ready-to-eat vegetable slices in your refrigerator. When these items are in front of you in the refrigerator, you'll gravitate toward them. If you put them in the bottom drawer, you'll forget they're there, and they'll spoil.

Picturesque kitchens speak a thousand words involving good health and a strong commitment to eating right. Post pictures of healthy living on your cell phone wall and on your computer. Hang an air freshener in the shape of a fruit from your rearview mirror and a shower curtain that contains fruits and vegetables on it. Get creative and bring wellness into your day, every day.

EXERCISES

(1) What pictures at home symbolize good health?

(2) What are two things I'll purchase this week to depict a healthy environment?

(3) What is a recent moment of truth (tool 17) where instead of turning to junk food for comfort, I chose something healthy instead?

TOOL 80. CREATE A DAILY AFFIRMATION

Set your intentions before you start every single day by deciding what you wish to do for yourself today. In other words, create your own daily affirmation and then live by it. Walk in the shoes of who you want to be. Put out positive energy into the universe about your weight-loss journey, and you'll be successful. Your personal affirmation can be, "I love being a fit and healthy person." Be specific with what steps you're taking to make this happen. No more negative thoughts regarding this journey, okay?

A client of mine e-mails me his daily affirmations since he loves sharing them with me. This is a client who is loaded with fire in his heart to succeed on his journey. He has been working with me for a short period of time, and because he keeps a daily journal, he is on top of his game. His affirmation right before New Year's 2012 was, "I feel like I've traveled for miles through a fog that is now slowly lifting. My intention for this week is to meditate on the things that truly make me happy." He is moving through challenges that have kept him mentally stuck. You get to paint the picture of the days you wish to live ahead.

Affirmations set you up for successful outcomes. There's no such thing as failing when the word failure isn't a part of your vocabulary. Hiccups or barriers may slow you down. It's how you handle these hiccups that makes you successful. Grooves in the road teach you how to build better traction. When you keep your eyes on your goal, you reach it in time. You are allowed to feel good about yourself and your life. Don't think otherwise.

My personal affirmation is "smile and believe." Smiling creates laughter and joy. Believing is knowing that there is no such thing as *can't*, *try*, or *fail*. Believing is knowing that you can. You must always believe in yourself no matter how hard something seems. You will always succeed when you work through it. Never quit. I also live by "If I can make one person laugh every day, then I've done a good deed." Laughter is medicine.

Let's put this into practice. Let's say you intended to work out today, but the day came and went. At night you find yourself sulking that you let yourself down by not exercising. Tomorrow, your intention will be "Through rain or snow, I will work out and nothing will stop me." When you choose a dynamic affirmation, it will motivate you to succeed.

Start off each week by saying, "Happy Monday!" to everyone you come in contact with. I love doing that. Monday is the beginning of a new week. A new week brings new opportunities for us. If you chose to not exercise three times last week, then make it happen this week. Monday is a gift. Don't repeat last week's behaviors if they didn't make you feel proud. Create an affirmation such as "I'm a fit individual, and I'm going to train three times this week!"

My grandma Sylvie's favorite affirmation is "I love myself." Grandma is eighty-eight years young, lives alone in New York City, gets around on her own, and is also writing a book. How? Because she can. Grandma told me that she was once 180 pounds back in the day. She now weighs 116 pounds. Living in a lean body keeps her mind and body full of life. How did she lose her weight? When she was in her late fifties, she joined Weight Watchers, which prompted her to make lifestyle changes. She changed her eating habits, decreased her portions, and became more active. Grandma claims that she performs water aerobics in the bathtub every day. I giggled when she told me this. I love her outlook on life and strive to be like her when I'm her age. She told me that she looks forward to living well into one hundred. If she keeps this up, she may live over 120 years.

EXERCISES

(1) What's my daily affirmation for today?

(2) What is one thing I did differently today that I'm proud of?

TOOL 81. LEARN SOMETHING NEW

If you're bored and dealing with the same old stuff, then you may be overeating out of complete boredom. Therefore, learn something new. New experiences bring new adventures. Writing this book was a new adventure for me. I feel amazing, and I know that I am going to feel even more amazing afterward by impacting the lives of millions of people (nothing wrong with putting it out there, right?) New opportunities can boost your self-esteem. A high self-esteem facilitates excellent behaviors that ultimately help you lose weight. It's crucial that you only take on what you can handle without sacrificing the original plan, a healthier you.

Consider taking one of the following classes:

- Nutrition seminar

- Sewing class

- Art class

- Bowling league

- A fundraiser involving fitness (Spinning, a 5K, or a walk-a-thon)

- Running clinic

- Sailing

- Salsa dance

- Swim lessons

- Tennis lessons

- Yoga workshops

I learn new things every year. For 2012, I got yoga certified through Tamal Dodge at the Yoga Collective in Santa Monica. This was a two-hundred-hour commitment which earned me the credentials of a registered yoga teacher through the Yoga Alliance. As much of a commitment as it was, I learned something new every day and met twenty four amazing people. And, would you believe that I learned how to perform a head stand? I never in my righteous mind would have ever thought that I can stand on my head. Thanks Tamal! It's empowering to get to learn something new every day of our lives. Look for those life lessons. It's up to you to ask questions so that you can learn all throughout your life. Make your life limitless!

TOOL 82. TRY ON YOUR CLOTHING

Make a date with yourself or with a friend on a Friday or Saturday night and create a fashion show. This tool serves two purposes. It allows you to unclutter your closet (tool 2), making room for smaller clothing. It also allows you to feel great about yourself again by taking *me* time to see what you've got. I did this with my mother when I was in New York once. She went through her closet as I sat on her bed. I remember she pulled out one garment at a time, displaying each item across her chest or hips. Some items were hideous, big, and some were even tight. If things were too big on her then I ordered her to donate them to charity. As she tossed items into the donation pile, she made a promise with herself that she'd never grow back into those big sizes again.

It's amazing how clothing is one of the best indicators for internal change. It's like a poster coming out of its poster sleeve. Have you ever taken out a rolled-up poster from the sleeve and tried fitting the poster back inside again? You probably struggled with the poster sleeve, as it seemed to have shrunk, even though it's exactly the same size as before. The objective is to reroll the poster until it fits inside the sleeve again. Parallel this to when you don't fit into your clothing. Even if you lie on your bed, jump up and down, or do side bends and silly maneuvers, it's always frustrating when fitting into your jeans is like fitting that poster into its sleeve. The worst is getting your skin caught in the zipper—ouch! To lose weight, you *must* tighten up your eating habits so that you can fit back into your sleeve again (and eventually into a smaller sleeve). When the sleeve gets too big, you get to size down, as seen in the next tool. Now that's what I'm talking about!

EXERCISES

(1) When will I put on a fashion show and try on my clothing?

(2) With whom, if anyone, will I do my fashion show?

(3) Where will I donate my old clothing?

TOOL 83. SIZE DOWN

After trying on your clothing, plan on sizing down one month later and go shopping. After consistently eating healthily, go to the mall and try on some clothing from affordable stores such as H&M, Forever 21, Target, Ross, and TJ Maxx. Your assignment is to shop once a month, and when you fit into the next size down from your current size, buy that article of clothing! Size down every step of the way. This will prove your progress.

I meet a lot of people who don't lose a lot of weight to start. The good news is that they lose inches and their clothes fit looser. This should be an awesome indication that you're doing great. This is why I don't want you to focus too much of your attention solely on the scale.

Weight-loss success can be seen through other changes, too. You can measure your body composition (tool 50) or your blood values (better cholesterol or lowered blood sugar levels). A patient I've been working with for two months only lost four pounds according to the scale. When we measured his body composition, however, we learned that he gained ten pounds of muscle and lost fourteen pounds of fat! Okay, different situation, wouldn't you agree? Losing weight is obviously the goal; however, consider measuring your success through other venues such as sizing down so that you can embody your success throughout your weight-loss journey. These additional variables will help you stay on track.

If you find the next size down doesn't fit, then take out your notebook and start writing in a journal (tool 28). Write down how much sleep you get each night, how much water you're drinking each day, what you're eating, and what type of exercise program you're doing. Get back to the basics because at the end of the day, if the basics become too loose, you'll plateau and you'll lose motivation. This doesn't mean you failed in your journey. Remember, failing isn't in your vocabulary. The goal of a journal is to take inventory of the things that need to change. The goal is to learn about the areas of opportunity within your journey so that you can strategize, set new intentions, and conquer the journey differently if need be.

EXERCISES

(1) What's the last size I purchased in the store?

(2) When will I go on my first sizing-down shopping spree?

(3) How will I track my sizing-down progress?

TOOL 84. PLAN A VACATION

Booking a vacation gives you something very exciting to look forward to for mental relaxation. A vacation also creates a new motivation to look your best. Your vacation may not be to a tropical island or to a place where you'll reveal a lot of skin, but think about this: if you're able to eat well and exercise regularly, then your vacation will be more relaxing. Why? When you're fit, your vacation becomes a relaxation tool as well as a vehicle for self-exploration. When you're unfit, vacations become a destination bed where you sit at a pool all day with a dozen cocktails and act lazy. Instead, be in a world that allows you to reflect on all the great things you've done prior to your trip. Vacations should not be about reflecting on how tired you are.

The average person takes approximately two weeks to settle into a state of relaxation while they're away. Why? My theory is because people take very little care of themselves these days, and this builds up an enormous amount of stress-related tension in their bodies. This tension causes physical exhaustion. Vacations are the time when our bodies slow down from going one hundred miles per hour to zero miles per hour. Vacations are when we actually feel the aftermath of our busy and stressful lives. In today's economy, many people aren't taking a full two-week vacation and therefore don't have enough time to settle into their abyss of pure relaxation. You're better off changing your lifestyle when you're home so that your body and mind can manifest an invigorated feeling for when you're on vacation. Vacation planning will serve you with urgency to make this change immediately.

Taking care of yourself will give you energy to spend quality time with your partner because you feel so great about life. This type of vacation is always a true reward. You'll find yourself remaining active through hotel activities and perhaps taking an early morning yoga class. A fit lifestyle also means never feeling embarrassed about how you look in photos either. Come on. Join me in living the lean lifestyle. It's such a better world. You will see!

EXERCISES

(1) Where can I go away on vacation?

(2) When can I go away on vacation?

(3) What will I do to ensure I get fit and relaxed for my trip?

TOOL 85. PLAN A PHOTO SHOOT

Hire a photographer for a photo shoot and schedule it six months from today. Decide on the location, what you'll wear, and what your end goal is for doing the shoot. Will it be on the beach, in a ballroom, at

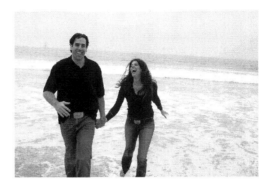

a gym, or in your own backyard? The goal of the photo shoot is simple. If you know you're hiring a photographer to take pictures of you, don't you think you're going to get into the best shape you possibly can? Six months is plenty of time to lose enough weight and inches so you can see a tremendous change in your body when you see the photos.

No matter how shy you are, have fun with this experience. Consider hiring a student from a local university or art school who wants to make a couple of dollars and practice photography. You can also consider a photo shoot with friends and split the cost for a professional photographer. Gather several families together for a shoot that involves your family *and* friends. Use these photos as your holiday cards or to simply show your progress every few months. The goal is to look your best for this shoot. Six months of excellent nutrition and ample levels of physical activity will gift you with a much leaner body than today.

I planned a photo shoot for my birthday this year with the amazing photographer Xochitl Rodrigue (she shot the photo for this tool). February is my birthday month, so it usually involves too much celebrating all month long. The shoot got Alan and me focused on looking our best for the photos. This deterred us from splurging. Good call, JZ! Photo shoots also give you experience in front of the camera. Imagine looking "hot" in family photos from now on! It's completely possible.

This photo shoot will also mark the beginning of an amazing transition period for you. It's almost guaranteed that you'll look great when you eat healthy and participate in physical activity before the shoot. I've used this tool with patients and it completely works. Four months prior to the shoot, I provided each participant with a *photo shoot* nutrition and exercise plan. How do you think models look great all the time? Because they participate in photo shoots all the time. No one said you have to be a model. But it's time to set the urgency factor high so that you live a healthy life today and every day.

EXERCISES

(1) When will I schedule the shoot?

(2) What will this photo shoot involve (costumes, location, people, cost)?

(3) Who will I invite to shoot with me?

TOOL 86. CREATE A VISION BOARD

A vision board is a very specific collaboration of goals, dreams, and desires you wish to achieve. First and foremost, allow your vision board to depict your goals for the year. Nothing happens overnight, which means your weight-loss goal can't be accomplished by tomorrow, unfortunately.

Your vision board should be a dynamic visual work of art that excites you and contains realistic goals. Some visuals that you can put on your board include the following:

- An image of an active person (perhaps of you)
- Your education, fitness, nutrition, career, and family goals
- Pictures of colorful vegetables to encourage healthy eating
- A relaxation photo for stress reduction
- A photo of your dream vacation destination
- A lean photo of yourself
- A reward for when you attain your goal weight

Let your vision board motivate you to achieve a healthy lifestyle. The more specific and realistic your goals are, the more motivated you'll be to do the work.

I recently reconnected with a former client of mine from almost two years ago. Not only has she gained back the eight pounds she lost (out of the forty she had to lose), but she also gained an additional ten pounds on top of that. I took her under my wing again and this time created a vision board for her. The vision board has a colorful pink background with photographs of footprints in the sand. For every five pounds she drops, she gets to place one footprint in the sand. Each footprint resembles one step closer to her end goal, which is going to Bora Bora in Tahiti. She only needs ten footprints to escape to Bora Bora. In the middle of the vision board is a photo of Bora Bora. This vision board is in her bedroom. She spends a lot of time with fit people, but they eat poorly around her. She joins them. Her body stores fat while her skinny friends don't. Why? Her body's physiology can't be compared to that of her lean friends because overweight individuals have different insulin sensitivities that stunt the utilization of fat when refined carbohydrates are consumed in excess. She must break her addiction to food (tool 15). She hired a home-delivery service that delivers food to her every day (tool 72). The vision board helps keep her on track while marking each milestone until she goes to Bora Bora.

Schedule a vision board creation day with your friends who also want to lose weight. Everyone should bring arts-and-crafts supplies, nice-looking boards, paint, fabric, magazines, and anything else that can go on the board. If everyone brings a healthy dish to this event, then everyone will also eat well. Remember, being healthy isn't simply about eating healthy. It's about creating an all-inclusive lifestyle that embodies an organic existence with a positive outlook.

EXERCISES

(1) What will be on my vision board?

(2) When is my first vision board meeting?

(3) Where will it be held?

(4) Whom will I invite?

TOOL 87. CREATE A WEIGHT-LOSS MASTERMIND GROUP

A mastermind group is a collaboration of many like minds with the same goal working as one group that shares best practices. Invite people you respect and wish to include in your weight-loss journey. Make sure these individuals are all on the same journey as you. The people you invite into the group can help you and each other break the chains of obesity once and for all by mastering the journey together. When people are surrounded by others who inspire them, positive outcomes can occur.

My friend Lisa Rainey facilitated a mastermind group called The Artist's Way with her friends, all of whom craved professional growth. *The Artist's Way* is a book that offers ambitious people the opportunity to successfully accomplish a creative goal by facilitating group meetings that create an urgency to do it. Lisa successfully arranged the group meetings, got people interested in attending, and created the themes for each meeting. She helped people move toward accomplishing their goals.

It makes perfect sense that people are more likely to succeed when they're surrounded by like minds with the same mission. You can establish this by finding between three to five committed people, choosing someone's home to meet in, and taking the group through a successful weight-loss journey.

First things first. Make sure everyone owns my book (*Breaking the Chains of Obesity, 107 Tools*) so that you can all reference the tools in the book. Next, decide how long the journey will be. Pick a realistic time frame (tool 75) so people can commit. Next, select where and when the meetings will be held. Consistency keeps the retention rate high. Don't be too fluid with the schedule; otherwise, people will flake out. Teach your group about the importance of accountability through committing to a weekly mastermind meeting. Last, decide who the group leader will be. This person should possess good leadership skills and should also send out weekly e-mail reminders that contain positive affirmations, outlines of past group discussions (a note-taker should type it up), and fitness, nutrition, and lifestyle tips.

Start off every meeting with a mission so everyone knows what to expect. Each person must find ownership in this mission. Keep it open for discussion. Go around and have each person share a weekly moment of truth (tool 17) with the group. Afterward, consider taking the group for a twenty-minute brisk walk or practicing yoga.

Here's a sample agenda of what you can do in your weight-loss mastermind group:

Week 1

The first week is a meet-and-greet. Sit in a circle and ask everyone to write down answers to some of the following questions:

- What diets have you tried?
- What were the strengths and the weaknesses of each diet?
- Why did you stop that diet?
- How much weight do you want to lose?
- How long have you been trying?
- What specific time frames do you wish to establish?
- What are your fears?
- How many times have you failed at dieting?
- Why have you failed at weight loss in the past?
- What is your biggest motivation today?
- How long have you been overweight?
- What is the most you have ever weighed?
- What is your optimal weight and how long ago was that?

- Is your spouse supportive of healthy eating?

- Are your children overweight? Siblings? Parents?

- Do you have health issues?

- Do you have joint issues?

- Do you take medications?

- How are your sleep patterns?

- What do you hope to get out of the mastermind group?

Go around the room and have everyone answer each question. Make this a comfortable experience. People can pick and choose what they share with the group. People should never feel uncomfortable or judged by this group. This should feel like a safe haven. Make this a dynamic discussion. Brainstorm strategies so that people can learn new methods of overcoming the hiccups that have stopped them before. Get to know each other. Learn to support each other no matter where everyone is in their weight-loss journey. The common goal is *mastering a lean lifestyle*.

Take a before picture of each participant and measure their weight, body fat percentage and all circumference measurements (chest, arms, abs, waist, hip, and legs.) Be sure to measure in the same spots each time. Consider hiring a personal trainer to do this part for you.

Week 2

Each person should create a vision board. See tool 86.

Week 3

Participate in a physical-fitness challenge. Hire a qualified personal trainer to ensure proper form and execution. Test each person on the following: push-ups, crunches, planks, squats, jumping jacks, lunges, and single-leg balances. Afterward, go around to each person and discuss what type of physical activity they participated in during the week. Learn a new fit tip from the trainer, too.

Week 4

Each person should research a healthy recipe, bring in a dish, and educate everyone about it.

Week 5

Identify the tools from *Breaking the Chains of Obesity* that resulted in successful outcomes for the group so far. Come up with a list of the top-ten tools each person is using and go around the room. If you recognize a tool that someone is successfully using but is a challenge for you, then write down your questions and conduct a brief Q&A session afterward. Interview each person after they're done speaking. Strategically position your question so you can get an answer that's meaningful for you and the group. Tell the group to check in to www.JZfitness.com each week so that new ideas are fostered for discussion.

Week 6

Bring in a mind/body coach or yoga teacher for ten dollars a person. If there are five people then fifty dollars is a great start for a yoga teacher who's looking to expand his or her business. It's time to relax and decompress. Ask this teacher to share the fundamentals of building a manageable meditation practice and also how to incorporate stress reducing techniques into your life on a daily basis.

Week 7

Demonstrate moment-of-truth (tool 17) skits in front of each other. Pair up with another person and make up a scenario to act out in front of the others. When you role-play a "dieting" struggle, you're able to *see* a familiar struggle and how others deal with it. As a group, discuss how each character handled his or her struggle. Role-playing allows people to visualize what they actually look like in a complicated situation. I learned this in college when I worked for Middle Earth Peer Education, founded by Dr. Dolores Cimini through the University at Albany. We enacted real campus behaviors, which emotionally connected the audience to the characters. The goal was to *mirror image* the behaviors and then plan strategies for change.

Week 8

Take an updated photo of yourself: front, side, and back pictures. Take new measurements. In a group discussion, share your overall experience from the last eight weeks. Everyone is in this with you. Reflect, respond, and feel the level of support you deserve.

These weekly meetings should facilitate true intentions for change. Find a streamlined focus, and it will benefit everyone involved. Be creative. Keep these meetings dynamic, and don't waste time during them. Keep everyone focused on why you're all there. This isn't a social hour. These meetings are meant to be productive so everyone can lose weight once and for all!

EXERCISES

(1) Who can I invite into my weight-loss mastermind group?

(2) When will I send out an e-mail invitation? (Blind cc all the people on your list just in case they don't want to share their personal information with others they don't know. Once you establish who's interested, send out the information to everyone regarding the first meeting.)

Here is a sample e-mail:

To all my special friends,

As you may know, I'm ready to lose weight. I have made countless attempts before, but now I'm ready! I would love for you to join me. At some point, you've told me that you wanted to lose weight as well. Is this still true? I know for a fact that if we do this together, we can help each other succeed. I propose that if we can congregate each week in a small group, we will all succeed at losing weight. I call it the weight-loss mastermind group. Please look at your schedule over the next week and let me know what days and times work for you. The location is to be determined. It will

be a private meeting for those I've chosen to help assist me
with this very sensitive goal. I love you so much and would
love to have you on my team. You can call me to get more
details about this mastermind group if you'd like. I look for-
ward to your reply.

Yours in good health,

Your name

Phone number

E-mail address

TOOL 88. WRITE A BOOK

A book can begin as an outline and develop into a string of
words that accidentally turns into a story. Have you ever considered writing about your own personal weight-loss journey?
Don't be scared to do so. Go to the dollar store and simply
purchase a spiral-bound notebook to write in. Start this journey
off by writing daily journals (tool 28). Eventually, you'll con-
solidate all your journal entries into a book at which point you
can choose to publish or not. If you do choose to publish, you
will possess strong credentials since you succeeded at losing
weight. This experience will allow you to share your experience with others who strive to lose weight, too. This can also
motivate you to stay on track each day since you know someone will be reading it someday. Your journals can be a big help
to someone.

Below is a daily journal template:

- Date

- My intentions for today

- My daily quote

- Nutrition section (write out each meal you ate)

- Exercise

- Moment of truth from today (tool 17)

- Any struggles

By *seeing* your actions in your journal, you can identify which behaviors are working and which are not. For example, if you look back to find that you haven't eaten enough vegetables, then you can add more vegetables into your day moving forward. You may realize you're not stretching enough or eating small, frequent meals. On a positive note, you can also see vast improvements in your behaviors now compared to a week or two ago.

Publishing a book can teach others how to apply the same tools you used to succeed. It's very rewarding to help other people break their chains of obesity. In all of my years of working in weight loss, I find that weight-loss students get motivated by other losers. The world needs more autobiographies out there so that breaking the chains of obesity can be a strong movement through successful storytelling. Your book can illustrate the trials and tribulations you faced in your journey and the tools you picked up along the way. You can write about the changes you've made in your everyday behaviors. It's a gift to share this with others.

You can write about the following topics:

- The barriers you faced

- What you did to overcome these barriers

- What set you back

- How you leaped forward

- How you felt throughout the process (day to day)

- How you instilled positive self-talk

- How you avoided saboteurs

- How you managed your stress

- How you managed your time

- How you fought the fears

- Anything else you "felt" along the way

There are published authors out there who have experienced the same journey that you did. I thank Charles Ciccarelli, who wrote *Life Is a Fat Onion,* a book that explains how he lost 155 pounds and what life is like today as a lean man. This book is a tearjerker. Perhaps reading it can help you in your weight-loss journey. It can certainly help you in your book-writing journey! Be inspired by Charles's book and write your own. Start with an outline of the chapters you wish to write. Then take the outline and write away. For example:

- Chapter 1: How I became overweight

- Chapter 2: How I discovered that I had to change

- Chapter 3: The major roadblocks I will face

- Chapter 4: Falling off track and getting back in the saddle again

- Chapter 5: Halfway to goal

Get the drift? Writing a book offers you the true intentions to simply do it. If you know you'll be sharing your journey with the world someday, you're going to feel an intrinsic force of desire to stay on course. Ever since I started writing this book, my grandma Sylvie told me that she admired me for writing a book and wished she could write one too. Can you believe that I convinced her to follow through with this wish? At the age of eighty-eight, grandma Sylvie is writing her own biography, which documents all of her life experiences. She lived through wars, the Great Depression, and other life events that helped make her the strong lady she is today. She has witnessed the evolution of our society and broke her chains of obesity more than twenty years ago. She has the sharpest mind I've ever known, and her ability to recollect the fine details of all her life experiences is extraordinary. This is the key to healthy aging. Even though she never knew she would actually write a book, she always told me that she should write a book about all she's been through. And so, I've convinced her. This is my little secret to keeping her young since I want her to be around for a long time.

EXERCISES

(1) When will I begin my book? (Create an outline and/or daily journal.)

(2) What will I name my book?

TOOL 89. DICTATE YOUR THOUGHTS

I sometimes drift off into the deepest of thoughts, and I like to capture these thoughts by recording them as they're happening in my mind. This is the artist in me. When creative juices start flowing, it's time to bring out the canvas. My canvas is my day. Getting a voice recorder allows me to record my ideas, goals, strategies, and thoughts before I forget them. Audio dictations provide more information, such as my tone of voice, accentuations of certain words, and the spontaneity of thoughts. You don't capture this on paper. The best news is that Best Buy and Amazon sell digital recorders for as low as forty dollars.

Let's call these recordings your own personal dictations. By transferring information out of your mind, you actively succeed at uncluttering your head! Record your voice throughout your weight-loss journey and use your dictations to write your book. How cool would it be if you had dictations of your entire journey? This can help you recall how you reached your goal. Don't you think you'll learn something new about yourself by doing this?

If you don't know how to start dictating, then simply pick a topic and practice. Write out a list of topics to talk about, and then just talk. For example, you can talk about how you feel about recording your voice. Talk about your realization of the need to change, your desire to be lean, your exercise program, or your moment of truth for the day. Discuss what you've learned from this book and comment on how these tools affect you. Talk about the *hiccups* that have veered you off path and how you will avoid them in the future. Dictations can provide you with valuable insight.

Record your journey so that you can learn how to survive the rocky roads and make a turn onto smoother roadways. You'll be amazed when you play back and hear how you've personally developed during this journey of change.

EXERCISES

(1) Do I own a recording device? If not, where will I purchase one?

(2) What topics can I talk about?

TOOL 90. SAY "I LOVE MYSELF" EVERY DAY

My grandma Sylvie taught me to recite this statement to myself. Over time, this has convinced me to love the person I am for who I am. I have learned to fall deeply in love with the little girl inside of me while evolving as a human being in the hectic world we all live in. As a result of self-love, I enjoy the depths of life including new venues, learning, feeling great, meeting new people, being a fitness guru, sharing my love with others, and teaching people about the beauty of life. I've tapped into a very spiritual side which better serves me. Since changing my outlook over time, my life has become one precious gift to me.

I've pledged to always be a good person. I am loyal, honest (sometimes too honest), and very lovable. When you think about yourself, find a way to be in love with who you are today by picking the top three traits you love about yourself. I know you don't like the weight you're at right now, so don't focus on that. In time, you will peel those layers off. The core person that is right within you today is the part you should find love for. That core person is the only one who will get you through this journey.

Start peeling off one layer at a time by using the tools in this book. Learn how to live inside of your body and not so much on the outside. Tune out all the external stimulants that prevent you from exploring your own inner beauty and light. Learn to conquer each barrier that held you back in the past, and realize that by conquering all your barriers today, you will strengthen the warrior within you and lose your weight.

The first step is to simply say out loud, "I love myself!" It may sound silly to say this, but the more you say it, the sooner you'll believe it. I conclude all of my Spin classes by having my students say, "I love myself." Why? Because they should. Loving yourself means wanting the best for yourself, taking care of yourself, and holding yourself to a high level of self-regard. Loving yourself allows you to be there for others. Love yourself for listening to others, for showing up to the gym, for helping someone out, or for taking them to the airport when they need a ride. Love yourself for everything you do for others. Self-love makes the world go around. Learn to love yourself no matter what you weigh right now.

Let's parallel your view of your vehicle to how you view your body. If you don't like your vehicle, you can vacuum it, put it through a car wash, get new floor mats, and even get a pink fuzzy steering wheel—just kidding! But do you see what I'm saying? You learn to work with what you've got. Do the same with your body. Learn how to make the best of what you've got while being at your current weight. Over time, you'll evolve into a more desirable weight through loving yourself.

Here are some ways you can show some love for yourself right now:

- Wear clothing that fits you reasonably well and isn't old, torn, or stained.

- Brush your hair.

- Try a new hairstyle or makeup.

- Try a new clothing style to accentuate your best features.

- Clean your car.

- Clean your desk.

- Write a poem or song.

- Pick something to do in this book today.

- Do a random act of kindness (tool 107).

Loving yourself allows you to treat your body like royalty. Loving your body means feeding it with healthy food. Move past the fear of failing, boredom, or feelings of isolation. It's time for a different script. The sooner you stop stressing about your weight and start embracing the lifestyle of a healthy person, the sooner you'll lose your weight. It takes patience and constant belief in yourself.

Look at yourself in a new light during this journey. Be in love with yourself right now. Think about all the goodness you bring into this world. Don't wait until you hit your goal weight before you start loving yourself. People will be more attracted to you. Whenever my Grandma roams the streets of New York City, people stop her to tell her how beautiful she is. The amount of love she feels for herself permeates the air. People want a piece of her positive energy. Her positive energy stems from self-love.

EXERCISE:

(1) Say, "I love myself!" out loud.

(2) What are some of my strengths and positive attributes?

(3) What will help me love myself today?

(4) Who are three people who are the closest to me? Ask them to state their top three reasons for loving me.

TOOL 91. RECORD YOUR WEIGHT-LOSS JOURNEY

Some people post their journeys on YouTube or Facebook. Videos capture your full expression.

On your video documentary, consider talking about how your days are. How have you progressed? What have you learned? What are your intentions for the day? Record your response to your struggles, which tool(s) you're using, how they worked or didn't work, how you will do things differently in the future, what you are proud of today, what you are not so proud of today, who your support system is, and what your affirmation is for the day.

Here's how you do it. Set up your camera or cell phone camera on a tripod or on a stack of books. Position yourself in front of the camera in a chair. Talk to the camera about the following:

- What are your name, age, and weight?

- What made you decide to lose weight?

- How many times have you tried before?

- What have you tried?

- What are you scared of?

- Do you enjoy physical activity?

- How did you get to your current weight?

- What has been holding you back from losing weight?

- What is your goal?

- Do you have any saboteurs in your life?

- What will you do to get around these saboteurs?

I have heard horrific stories about how parents don't believe in their child's weight-loss journey. It's hurtful, I know. But it's your life. Ask yourself how you want to live it. Are there cultural barriers in your way? What barriers do you face? Narrate all of these situations on your video, and begin developing a plan of action so that you can address these obstacles.

When you're ready, you may choose to mail your footage to a place that will edit your video for you. My friend Brock has a great company called *Memens* in Newport Beach, California. They professionally film and edit videos of the older population but will provide video for virtually anyone who wants to capture their own personal journey. It's amazing to watch your journey blossom into a home video that tells a tremendous story about your success.

A documentary also allows you to reflect on your journey. The goal is to learn from your past so that you can forever love your life and the body you're living in moving forward. The goal is to keep your weight off forever.

EXERCISES

(1) When will I use the above documentary guidelines and begin creating my video?

(2) Which setting makes me feel comfortable enough to be as real as possible for my video?

TOOL 92. GO THROUGH OLD PICTURES

Allow yourself to reminisce about the past chapters of your life. If this is a sore subject for you, awesome! You must think I'm crazy for saying that, but photos can dig up the deepest, most suppressed memories that you should deal with today. When you identify the things that bothered you in the past and still bother you now, you can unclutter your mind of those things and lose weight. So, if it means finding peace and forgiveness for the people who have caused you pain in the past, then do it. Stop wasting your energy by feeling angry. Or, if you lost touch with a close friend and that has played on your mind, reach out to him or her and fill the void you've felt for years.

Pictures allow you to relive the memories of certain points in your life that touched you both mentally and emotionally. If you're not happy with where you are today, it's time to change. Pictures can represent where you wish to go. For example, one of my patients showed me photos of himself from ten years ago when he and his wife wore skintight action figure Halloween costumes. He claimed that those were the most fun times in his life. I told him to keep those photos handy during his weight-loss journey. They encourage him to eat well and exercise each week so that he can fit into those costumes again soon. This has been working great for him.

If photos are truly too painful for you to look at, then don't take this journey alone. Consider finding an external source to help you overcome the issues of your past to help you find peace of mind in the present.

EXERCISES

(1) When I look at past photos of myself, what are my initial thoughts?

(2) What behaviors must I change today that I got away with back then?

TOOL 93. RECONNECT WITH A FRIEND

Wouldn't seeing a past friend motivate you to look your best? This person should be someone who resembles a time in your life that you had a different mindset and a high self-esteem. I'm not talking about a person who made you feel crummy all the time or the date who dumped you just before the prom. I'm talking about a person you know will go nuts over seeing you. Building up the anticipation of seeing someone from your past might help to drive you back on track with healthier behaviors.

Once we graduate high school, we unfortunately separate from the people we grew up with by attending different universities. You naturally lose touch with most of your high-school friends unless you continue to reside in the same hometown the rest of your adult life or go to the same college. This happened to me, especially once I moved three thousand miles away from my hometown.

Then along came Facebook. When Facebook first came out, everyone asked me, "You don't have a Facebook account?" Their question was spoken in tones of extreme awe, like I was an outcast or something. So I signed up. Peer pressure once again. After getting an account, Facebook reconnected me with all those awesome people from my past. I even put together a JZ fitness fan page so that people can access my blog posts more conveniently.

Let me share a great story with you. I made plans to go to coffee with a former high school friend, Theresa Castaldo, whom I hadn't seen for fifteen years. Growing up, I had a lot of respect for Theresa. She was an athlete, she was beautiful, popular, and just a great girl.

There's significance to this story. Right before her reaching out to me, I spent five weeks fighting a terrible cold virus and sinus infection and ate cookies virtually every single day. I reverted back to being a little girl again when I was terribly ill. I needed inner comfort and an escape from feeling like utter crap every day! (So learn from my mistake: when you're sick, do not eat sugar, drink juices, or eat sweets. If you do, it's like sending your virus to the playground; it will keep you sick longer. You will get better quicker when you stick to low glycemic eating.) I definitely needed a reason to stop eating cookies. Having plans with Theresa redirected my focus back to eating well again.

Calling a friend to debrief (tool 20) about your day is a better source of motivation compared to turning to food for comfort. Having someone to talk to can prevent you from eating something that only soothes you in the moment. Don't be a complainer by any means. Bounce ideas and situations off your friends by getting their insight on things. Choose to surround yourself with friends who are health conscious and invested in your weight-loss journey with you. A good friend will offer you the emotional support you need.

EXERCISES

(1) Whom should I reconnect with?

(2) What is a realistic amount of weight I should lose before seeing them?

(3) Whom can I call if I need to talk to someone?

243

TOOL 94. WATCH THE SUNSET

In life, we have good days, great days, and of course, bad days. However, the one thing we're blessed with every day is a sunrise and a sunset. Seldom do we stop in our day to respect what Mother Nature provides us with. Find a sunset and dive into it. Allow this beautiful sunset to do the following for you:

- Dump the stressors of your day into the sunset so that tomorrow brings better momentum for you.

- Reflect back on what you did today versus what you didn't do today.

- Thank your source of power for the opportunity to make the necessary changes to lose weight and for the tools that lie within you.

- Count the colors in the sky and determine that same number of moments of truth you experienced today (tool 17).

- Call one person you haven't called for a while, and tell them you love them.

- Focus on deep breaths as you exhale all the bad energy out of your body allowing room for a new breath of light.

Close your day with peace and serenity, and just know that you did your very best to be your best today. You can only look back and celebrate the greatness of today. Sunsets are magical memoirs of another successful day on this planet in good health and hopefully in good spirits. Don't take this for granted. It's seriously up to you to give energy back to yourself after a long day of giving your energy to others. You deserve to love yourself and be proud of who you are every day. Allow each step in this weight-loss journey to open up with a plan of action at sunrise and end with a prayer at sunset.

EXERCISES

(1) Where do I have access to a good sunset within ten miles of my home or work?

(2) How many colors were in the sunset?

(3) Which moments of truth did I reflect on?

TOOL 95. GO TO A HEALTH FAIR

Each year, major metropolitan cities host a public health fair. Health fairs are excellent venues to learn about the latest and most cutting-edge health advice out there. Health fairs usually have health screenings that check cholesterol, blood pressure, height, weight, and body composition.

Local hospitals, universities, wellness vendors, chiropractors, fitness professionals, lifestyle professionals, and insurance companies usually have booths at these fairs. The theme is preventative medicine. Do you realize that when you attend healthy events you gravitate toward healthier behaviors when you leave? I apply these same strategies when guests visit my home. I set up healthy games, prepare healthy food, and provide lifestyle lessons that educate people on being healthy. For example, my friend and her son came over, and I cut up little cucumber discs and spread low-fat cream cheese and salmon on them, and served them to him. Because her son is overweight and loves junk food, I wanted to teach him that healthy eating can also be yummy. He loved them.

Some companies offer health fairs to educate their employees about wellness and preventive medicine. When a company invests in its employees' health, employees become more productive and less sick during the year. If your company doesn't offer a health fair, perhaps you should initiate one. Lead by example. Being the leader of wellness will benefit your weight loss goal, too. Ask your CEO or HR representative if you can organize it. Keep it small to start. When I managed a health club, we had a two-day health fair and it was a tremendous hit. We brought in a variety of local vendors who aligned with health and wellness, including yoga apparel, natural jewelry, a health food store, a local chiropractor, a local hospital, supplement companies, and health-care providers. The members loved the opportunity to learn about new things and meet local vendors and health care professionals. So, be the leader (tool 100) that everyone needs. Set up a fun and exciting health fair to help break the chains of obesity in your neck of the woods.

EXERCISES

(1) Whom could I talk to in my company to organize a health fair?

(2) Where and when is the next health fair in my town?

TOOL 96. GO ON A RETREAT

Retreats are the time to reflect on your own intuition and withdraw from the stressors of everyday life while regenerating your vigor for a sound mind, body, and soul. Go with your favorite person, your spouse or a friend, or go alone if that works better. Retreats are offered through yoga studios, spa resorts, churches, temples, and spiritual centers. They are usually held in other countries or on exotic islands. I know my amazing yogi-girls Liz Arch and Jennifer Pastiloff host retreats each year. The best thing that I suggest you do is take a few classes from teachers who host retreats and if you like their energy, choose their retreat. Retreats allow you to reset your mind to a lighter tone of life filled with laughter, joy, physical activity, and good nutrition every day you're there. Retreats also offer the following benefits:

- Improved mental and physical health

- A jumpstart on your weight-loss journey with a healthy frame of mind

- Physical activity such as hiking, canoeing, kayaking, swimming, or yoga

- Healthy, organic nutrition that is calorically in alignment with what you need, prepared healthily, and cooked to taste yummy and wholesome

- A network of cool people who share common goals with you

- Learning how to meditate and actually relax

Some retreats offer leadership workshops. Many times, we lose the ability to lead ourselves through a healthy way of life simply because we exert too much energy in leading others. Efficient leadership skills will conserve your energy so there's energy left for you at the end of the day.

Part of losing weight successfully is putting your needs first. I use the airplane analogy. When you go on a plane, you hear the same safety instructions every time. The question is, do you ever listen to them? If you do, then do you remember the flight attendant stating that you must secure the oxygen mask over your face first before helping others? If you don't take care of yourself first in the event of an emergency, then you'll asphyxiate and won't be able to take care of anyone in the end. Use this analogy in your weight-loss journey. If you don't help yourself first, then your health will deteriorate, and in the end, you won't be able to help anyone.

I know you must be thinking that it's easier said than done. Everything in life is easier said than done. This is not a reason to ignore change. Putting yourself first means making time for your workouts, your meal preparation, and your mental downtime.

After you've met your own needs, then and only then should you avail yourself to others. Get in the habit of lending yourself to others rather than giving yourself to others. Give yourself to yourself. Don't put yourself in the backseat to the world. If your number-one goal is to make others happy, the formula for doing so is to take care of your body, mind, and soul first. People who love you want you to be happy. Your loved ones also want to see you in a good mood. When you're unhealthy, your mood can't be good because you're exhausted and stressed out.

A retreat can help you focus on what you need to do to keep your priorities aligned with your goals. Treat yourself to a getaway that teaches you how to reconnect with yourself.

EXERCISES

(1) Which retreat will I attend?

(2) Today, what was my moment of truth (tool 17) for putting myself first?

(3) Why is right now the best time to take a retreat?

TOOL 97. WRITE A PROMISE LETTER TO YOURSELF

Writing to-do lists (tools 1–4), help you create concrete and attainable goals. When you write things down, you "see" your intentions as you originally saw them in your mind. This makes your mission completely possible. Keeping goals and thoughts in your head doesn't always allow these goals to manifest into reality. Many ideas get lost in translation since thoughts turns sour, appear to be too much work or are simply forgotten altogether.

For this tool, I want you to pick out a theme and write yourself a promise letter. You don't have to write a report or think too much about the words you put on paper. The purpose of this letter is to commit yourself to a goal you really want. If you want to start with the obvious, then write yourself a weight-loss promise letter. When would this letter come in handy? For example, let's say that going to your mom's house for dinner always pushes you to eat the wrong stuff. This may never change. You must therefore have a solid plan of action in place in order to succeed. You will *always* be bombarded with choices. Form a plan of action that helps you face these challenges. You will be more successful when you do this.

Take control of your journey. You get to choose the food you eat, how much you eat, and when you'll eat it. For example, when you go to your family's house, your options are as follows:

- Avoid going

- Go and just eat what's there

- Eat a meal before you go so that you eat only a small amount when you're there

- Prepare your own dish to share with others

You have choices! Pick one that works for you. Write a promise letter to yourself as if you're coaching yourself through a tough situation. I've decided to draft a sample letter for your convenience. Your letter can look like the one below:

> *Dear Me,*
>
> *I am writing myself this letter to pledge my commitment to myself so that I can lose weight no matter what life tosses my way. I'm going to my mom's and I know that she's going to make a comment about my diet. She may even tell me that I lost too much weight already and that she's concerned about me. She and others will say, "Come on. It's only one day! We never get to see you. Mom worked hard on this casserole. Please don't offend her by being on your diet today."*
>
> *No matter what people say to me, I will commit to my plan. My plan is to eat before I go to the house so that I'm not starving. I will try a piece of Mom's casserole to be polite, but it'll be a very small portion. I will also bring something with me to show my love for my family. I will not talk about my diet with anyone when I get there. I will commit to being pleasant, and I will even leave at an hour that fits my schedule and plans.*
>
> *Respectfully yours,*
>
> *Myself*

Yes, I know, folks. It's a different approach for some of you and "cheesy" for others, but it can work very well. Take full accountability for your success. It's your job to take ownership of your actions and choose a road that works for you. No more pointing fingers at anyone else.

EXERCISES

(1) Which event do I need to write a promise letter for so that I can make it through successfully?

(2) What do I want to include in this letter?

TOOL 98. ACCENTUATE YOUR ASSETS

I always come across dieters who put themselves down. Stop putting yourself down—please! I know you have at least one body part that is extraordinary. Let's accentuate it. Don't think too hard about this one. Below, write down your favorite body part that makes you proud. Then, plan on accentuating this part forever by accessorizing it. For example, one of my clients has gorgeous hands. She always wanted to be a hand model. After having this conversation with her, she began taking better care of her fingernails and cuticles and presented silky, smooth hands that ultimately ignited her attitude. That was my goal with this tool.

I have another client whose hair is silky, shiny, and just stunning. She learned to accentuate her hair with the perfect earrings and outfits. Her hair is the first thing you see as a result. Even though she has fifty pounds to lose, she always shows up like a sexy woman because she has embraced her asset.

How about you long-legged ladies? If your abs aren't as tight as you'd like them, then show off your sexy legs instead. When you love yourself, you have an attitude that makes you so much more desirable to be around. People will be attracted to you if you focus on whatcha got versus whatcha don't got. If you want something that you don't have yet, then you must work for it. This is where working out is crucial.

A tight, lean body doesn't just come on a plate. It comes from committing to the lifestyle that makes it tight and hot! That commitment includes lifting weights, doing cardiovascular exercise, eating healthily, and possessing a positive mindset. A quick secret: lean people aren't always "into it." I personally get bored with the same routine, so I sometimes exhaust my muscles in thirty minutes or less. I do my cardiovascular exercise outside instead of on a piece of equipment. I sometimes hire a trainer. Mixing things up keep things exciting so that your boredom doesn't excuse you from a great workout. I eat very well and cheat only once in a while. A sample cheat for me is having two servings of pomegranate and vanilla cashews or cocoa cashews instead of one serving. Yup, my true confession! So, when people admire my lean body, I tell them that I work my tail off to look like this. And that's the truth.

Once you "get it," you'll be on a completely different level. My goal for writing this book is to teach you how to "get it." You must be the one to *do* the tools in this book. Adopt an "I can" attitude, and then just make it happen. Play up your assets. Self-empowerment begins with self-love so that you can be even better tomorrow.

EXERCISES

(1) What is my favorite body part?

(2) What will accentuate this body part?

(3) Which body part do I wish to improve?

(4) What is my plan to improve this body part?

TOOL 99. INTERVIEW A SUCCESSFUL LOSER

Remember in high school when you dreaded being called a loser? Well now you must love it, right? Ah-ha! I had a client say to me once, "I feel like such a loser." My response to her was, "You wish!" People who successfully lose weight are simply ready. They know what they need to change and are *willing to do whatever it takes* to get there. Remember, one day at a time. I know I keep saying this, but one day, you will seriously start doing this—if you haven't already.

Remember to keep mastering the first four tools. Always be conscious about the act of uncluttering. If you're looking to learn about new strategies to overcome the things that have obstructed your weight loss, then consider talking to someone who's been there and done it already. Your goal of talking to a loser is to learn about how they got through the tough times of change. This person should offer you a new perspective that perhaps you never considered.

A successful loser can also offer you hope. People tend to be inspired to change when they know their goal is attainable. Don't forget, the person you speak with was once in your shoes. Let's take a recent situation that happened between two of my clients. For confidentiality, I'll call them Bob and Bill. Bob came in one day right as Bill was leaving. It was perfect timing because Bill had lost twenty-two pounds of fat, and Bob had been struggling. At the end of fifteen minutes, Bob found a new breath of motivation through his conversation with Bill. Bill told him about his traveling schedule, how demanding his family life is, and how overweight he was. He told Bob to work through it and that everything will become easier—there's more energy for traveling and exercising on the road, energy and patience for his family, and a higher confidence in himself with his new physique. Thank goodness this conversation happened. Bob was close to quitting. You can't allow yourself to get discouraged, so talk to a loser.

Your success is an arm's length away. Your personal drive and motivation determine your outcome. Remember, you must decide every single day that you're not going to take any detours or long routes. The shortest distance is always that of a straight line, which is why staying on track will get you quicker results.

EXERCISES

(1) Whom will I interview about successful weight loss?

(2) What personal struggles do I wish to discuss with another loser?

TOOL 100. BE THE LEADER

Apply all the things you've learned so far in your weight-loss journey so that the world around you can follow. As a fitness expert, I can't break America's chains of obesity by myself. I need healthy leaders like you who can impact the people around you. Your leadership can facilitate change in your town and at your job. Being a leader will make your journey much easier, too. People need good leadership these days more than ever before. They will want to hang out with you because you'll be more energetic, fun, and in a great mood. This is what I call a synergistic relationship.

Leadership requires you to first identify who you are so that people know who they're following. You must live in the experience of what you'll be leading others to do. If you're cluttered with a million and one things to do, then teach those around you about the art of uncluttering.

Lead people through behavioral change by depicting what a healthy lifestyle looks like. You will continue to come up against certain barriers. These stumbling blocks are your lesson plans for your followers. It's up to you to learn how to overcome these barriers and teach your followers how you succeeded through any hiccups.

Leading others makes your journey very empowering. Realize that there's no such thing as failing when you simply commit to a healthier lifestyle. Here are some behaviors you can implement as the leader:

- Arrange filtered water at the office so everyone has access to water all day.

- Arrange an annual health fair.

- Pack your lunch every day.

- Arrange healthy food for corporate meetings.

- Start an office-wide daily affirmation.

- Ask others to join a gym with you under a corporate membership.

- Host a weight-loss contest within a time frame (twelve weeks) for a cash prize.

- Host a daily noon stretch at the office.

Being the leader requires you to care, be conscious, and be committed. This will create a sense of urgency to stay in control over your lifestyle behaviors since you know others are watching you.

EXERCISES

(1) As a leader, what's the first thing I'll do?

(2) Whom do I wish to lead?

(3) How can my personal journey impact them in a viable way?

TOOL 101. CREATE A WEIGHT LOSS BUCKET LIST

After watching *The Bucket List* with Jack Nicholson and Morgan Freeman, I had a tremendous aha moment. I always wondered why the very sick are the happiest people I've ever met, and why the healthy are usually not. When someone is given months to live, they immediately focus on the gratitude they feel for their loved ones and for the nonmaterial things in life. I find it interesting that more people don't create a bucket list while they have the rest of their lives to finish it. Dying shouldn't be our call to start living.

Be proactive in your journey. Create a weight-loss bucket list. This list is your own reward system that will motivate you to follow through with lifestyle changes. It should include the things you really want to have. Also include rewards you can't enjoy at your current weight. For example, when you lose your first ten pounds, you'll get a spa treatment. At twenty pounds, you'll go on a beautiful bike ride tour in wine country. At thirty pounds, you'll go on a shopping spree at your favorite mall. At forty pounds, you'll go away to a tropical island. For some people, a bucket list item is being able to chase after their grandkids. These are just examples.

I have bucket list items. For example, I always wondered how people conjured up the guts to step off a plane and sky dive. I always thought you had to be crazy to do this. I purchased tickets for my fiancé and me for his 2011 birthday gift. Yeah—a girl with a true fear of heights decided to take the leap of faith—literally. I went skydiving to conquer this fear. How did it go? Well, I'm obviously fine if I'm finishing this book, right? I remember the plane ride up to the ten-thousand-foot mark being a nerve-jerker for me, but I told the camera crew that if I could skydive, then I could do anything.

It's all about setting up dynamic goals for yourself and then following through with them. Don't just focus on the weight loss itself. How boring and dull. Using a bucket list makes life very interesting and bold. Do this with your weight-loss goal and even other goals. A bucket list is really just a dynamic goal sheet.

I would love to share more of my fun bucket list items with you to show you how great this concept really is:

- write a book (check—can't wait to write more)
- perform on stage (check)
- manage a health club (check)
- manage a medical weight-loss clinic (check)
- put together a charity event/one-woman act (check)

- get a master's degree in kinesiology or exercise science (check—I love education)

- live in Hollywood (check)

I could go on. Although my goals didn't pertain to weight loss, they still required a lot of work and perseverance to achieve them. One of my bucket list items is to own a wellness center one day. I keep my goals dynamic which makes my life fun and full of life. My bucket list items require a lot of time and energy, but in the end, they're all worth it.

What's your list going to look like? Allow this list to be full of mini rewards as you move toward your weight loss goal. I understand that being on a weight loss journey is a challenging road to travel. However, once you achieve your goal weight, you can do virtually anything in the world. Why? Because you accomplished a goal that's been a struggle for you for many years. This will prove that you can do whatever you put your mind to as long as you never quit.

EXERCISES

(1) What will I put on my bucket list?

(2) Which of these items will I concentrate on for this year?

(3) Other than weight loss, what is another long-term goal of mine?

TOOL 102. GO TO TEMPLE OR CHURCH

If you were raised in a place of prayer, then it would behoove you to go back to your roots and reconnect with your Creator. When we feel a sense of hopelessness, lost and alone in our journey, our creator is always there for us. I have friends and a grandmother who pray every day. I always admired their solid outlook on life. I finally got in touch with it again, and since then, my perception on life has been amazing.

How does religion help you in life? I must mention Eugene, an employee at the United States Post Office. No matter how nasty customers are to him, Eugene has a sense of centeredness that I admire. I asked him the other day how he manages to remain so positive despite all the negative attitudes thrown his way each day. His exact words were, "Girl, I thank Jesus every day for my serenity. My life is always in the hands of Jesus so I never let people get to me!" He never lets his customer's attitudes bring him down. Eugene goes to church every Sunday.

Another inspiration is the passionate work of Rabbi Chaim Mentz from the Chabad of Bel Air. Rabbi Mentz provides Torah entertainment, which offers Jewish people a light and entertaining twist on the Torah and how to reconnect to religion. He is nonjudgmental and truly loves all humanity. He's patient and focused on getting people reconnected to G-d. He has changed many lives.

When life seems unbearable, consider gathering in a place of prayer. Allow this experience to lead you. Spirituality will enhance your emotional intelligence so that you can succeed through life's biggest challenges. You won't need bad food to get you through tough times when you learn to choose healthier outlets. You no longer need to lie to yourself or to your weight-loss coach about your behaviors each day. Avoid cheating on your plan. Be real with yourself so that you can move past the shameful rationalizations and denial.

Stop saying you're too busy. It's up to you to make the time and ditch the "I'm too busy" excuse by prioritizing your life. Start saying, "I need to connect with my spiritual side so that I can alleviate all unnecessary stress in my life." Take one step at a time and go once or twice a month to your sanctuary of choice. Put it on your calendar. If religion is not your thing, then perhaps a spiritual center like the Agape International Spiritual Center is better for you. Some people even choose yoga to reach a spiritual place. Either way, choose the road that will help you achieve your goal.

EXERCISES

(1) What place of prayer will work best for me?

(2) What have I tried before?

(3) Has it worked before? If not, why?

TOOL 103. DON'T COVER UP ANYMORE

I've worked with so many people who wear big outfits to cover bloat and fat. You realize that the bloat will go away once you change your eating habits and begin to exercise, right? Rather than hide from the world, change your lifestyle behaviors and step out into the open world of endless opportunity for personal development.

Don't be scared! If you're used to wearing big clothing that hides you, then it's time to come out of hiding and shed those outer layers. This allows you to face the truth and work toward melting away the inside layers. Talk about symbolism. This tool truly defines the meaning of shedding your fears, sorrows, and weight so that you can be the lean person you deserve to be.

After uncovering, you will see yourself. Once you see yourself, you'll embrace who you are and find the urgency to take action. No matter how much you weigh, stop hiding. Hiding will keep the weight on your body. If you don't see it, you won't think about it, right? Not a good thing. So if you wear baggy sweats and baggy sweatshirts, start off by changing your baggy sweatshirt to a cute tee. You can even wear lululemon pants and a baggy shirt.

People are most self-conscious about their stomachs. To get over your fear of exposing more of yourself, consider taking a belly-dancing class. I learned belly dancing from my friend Brandi Reed, who is amazing at it. She has no shame in just pulling up her shirt wherever we are, exposing her abs, and gyrating her belly to any beat out there. Not only is she talented and beautiful, but she remains in tune with her body. Brandi can have five extra pounds on her, but it'll never stop her from showing some skin.

As an overweight person, you need to shed the layers of shame and protection. To do that, you must dump the fears that cause you to hide. Fear hasn't worked for you in the past. Fear has kept the weight on you for all these years. Look in the mirror, know who you are, and plan on making those changes. Embrace your body for what it is today. It will change in due time.

EXERCISES

(1) Is there a layer of clothing that I can shed?

(2) How will I become comfortable with the idea of not covering up?

(3) Where will I try a belly dancing class?

TOOL 104. SHADOW A TRAINER FOR A DAY

When people admire a trainer's body, most people don't realize that it took years of hard work to look as hot as they do today. I find that there aren't many people who have a clue about what healthy living means. Some trainers, like my friends Big Will, Ralph Remy and Hedda Royce, compete in shows to stay super lean. Other trainers like to maintain a lean physique without the "shredded" look. Pick a trainer you wish to follow so you can see how they do it. You get to witness a trainer's behaviors on a typical day and learn how trainers get to be super fit. The only thing that won't be typical in the trainer's day is they probably won't train their clients when you shadow them. Most clients don't want an outside person watching them workout. You can ask them about this.

I will warn you that shadowing a trainer will cost you for their time. Perhaps you can barter a service with them or treat them to a day's worth of meals. Work something out because trainers usually train clients, so if they're going to teach you some valuable lessons instead of train people, the price tag on their time is worth considering.

Let's take a typical day for me. I wake up after seven hours of good sleep, take my vitamins, pack my cooler with all my food for the day, drink twelve ounces of water, drive to work, coach people in weight loss, get my afternoon work- out in (it varies each day), go home, leave again to train or teach a class, and then go home and cook for tomorrow. I go to bed no later than ten thirty p.m., depending on the night. This lifestyle takes a strong commitment to myself and excel- lent organizational skills.

Organization is key, which is why I wrote the first four tools in this book. No matter who you are, you must remain uncluttered to be successful. I have learned that leading a very stressful life will only make you sick. Self-work is some- thing that requires a conscious state of being every single day. You don't mind the work since it makes you feel good about yourself and about life. The work never ends.

Create your own way of life and then live by it. If you don't want to be fat, then stop behaving like a fat person. Ask your trainer which of your behaviors constitute as fat behaviors so that you know. Once you know them, begin to change them. Take on the trainer's behaviors. Treat this opportunity like a big stage so you can truly experience the life of the most fit people out there—personal trainers. Remember, there's no such thing as failing. Being a coachable person will allow you to acquire the body you want. Just be patient. Use this experience as a lesson plan for mastering a healthier journey. There's nothing more powerful than playing the role of a successful loser. Once you become a loser, you'll transition over into being a winner in the end.

EXERCISES

(1) Whom can I shadow?

(2) What are three tools I wish to master with the trainer?

(3) What are the top ten questions I have for this trainer?

Chapter 5

HUMANITARIANISM CAN LIFT YOUR SOUL

Part of giving back as a humanitarian is being kind and offering your time, effort, and sometimes money to those in need. These missions introduce you to the immaterial side of life, where in most cases, people don't even have a home or access to fresh food and water. In your weight-loss journey, giving back to less fortunate individuals will bring positive energy into your life. Being a humanitarian reminds you that life is immaterial. Life is actually a gift that should never be taken for granted. This life lesson helps a lot of people move forward through any of life's challenges, even if your challenge is losing weight.

TOOL 105. VOLUNTEER

Volunteering gives you an immense amount of appreciation for humanity. There's a collaboration of love and generosity at charitable events. How great can that make you feel? The best part—money is left out. Volunteering instills a higher level of self-worth in you because your time is that valuable and you're lending it to others. When you feel good about what you've done, you love yourself more and respect your time more. Simply being a good person and sharing the wealth of your time and love with those in need is priceless.

Your weight-loss success stems from your ability to find motivation and purpose from within you. If you're not feeling motivated and need a new purpose, then becoming a volunteer can help you. Volunteer at a local town hall or church. Teach group exercise classes to individuals who can't afford a gym membership. Consider organizing a class such as boot camp, dance, or aerobics through a local school so that you and others can exercise. Local hospitals and nursing homes are also looking for solid volunteers. Did you know that many patients don't get visitors? When a sick patient doesn't have visitors, their desire to live eventually declines. As a volunteer, you can give that patient a purpose to live.

There are also humanitarian efforts both on our homeland and overseas that always need dedicated volunteers. Natural disasters are mostly to blame. There are many organizations to choose from. Do a Google search online and pick an organization that works for you. I imagine the Red Cross can always use an extra hand. I volunteered with the Red Cross after 9/11, helping to make beds and provided emotional support for those who were involved in clean up at ground zero. These efforts took place out of New York Sports Clubs on Wall Street. As sad as that experience was, I know that my love and help were very much appreciated, which helped me to mentally get through my losses from that disaster.

Some people may be at a point in their lives when they feel like they're giving a little too much, leaving little to no time for themselves. If this is you, then consider donating to a charity instead. Only volunteer at the level you are able to healthily do so.

EXERCISES

(1) Which organization do I wish to volunteer for?

(2) If I do not have the time to volunteer, which humanitarian efforts will I engage in?

(3) What will the benefit of volunteering be for me?

TOOL 106. DONATE TO CHARITY

Make it fun: go door-to-door and tell each neighbor that you're raising money for a half-marathon where all proceeds will go to a charity (find a date within six months and a charity you wish to walk/run for.) Tell your donors that your goal is to raise a certain amount of dollars for every mile you complete. You will be so surprised to see how many people donate money and how this can turn out to be a winning situation for the charity (they make money) and for you (it feels great to help) while training for an active event (fitness, baby!)

The best time to donate to charity is when you feel like you need more money. Donating a little of what you have reminds you of those who are less fortunate, and it will find its way back to you in some form. Find the fulfillment in giving another human being a little piece of what you've got, and revert back to the immaterial side of life. Even though you're donating money, which is technically material, you're actually putting less emphasis on possessing more money yourself by sharing it with others. You should only donate what you can, and there is no law about how much that is. Some people will donate nothing because they feel that nothing is better than a small amount. This isn't true.

Danny Thomas from St. Jude Children's Research Hospital stated that if ten thousand people donated a dollar, then it would add up to ten thousand dollars for the charity. He stated that he would rather have ten thousand people donating a dollar rather than one person donating ten thousand dollars. The power of teamwork has made his foundation a successful one. Remember, the little bit that you can give goes a long way for charities.

If you have more time, consider organizing a charitable function, too. I'll never forget having tea with my friend Adam Reid back in September 2010 when he dared me to perform in a one-woman act show. I told him that I didn't have any time to be involved in a performance right now. *Having no time* is the most common excuse I hear from those who don't want to prioritize exercise and food preparation during their weight-loss journey. So, how in the world was I going to use the *I have no time* excuse and not pursue something I love?

I decided to make a statement by taking this challenge on. I woke up my Grandma at one a.m. (New York time) to tell her to book a flight to Los Angeles for my birthday show. After screaming for joy in a half-awoken state, Grandma asked me what the show was about. I told her that it was a surprise (simply because I had no clue myself). I decided to make the show a charitable event and raised money for St. Jude Children's Research Hospital by charging twelve dollars a ticket. This event got me back on stage and allowed all of my LA friends to hear me sing.

I had many generous donors: the Ledson Winery in Sonoma, California donated wine; Whole Foods donated food and gift cards, Canters Deli donated birthday cookies, D-Roc donated music, 220 Fitness donated two memberships, Robert Rivera donated photography, Michael Schweitzer donated videography, and Negotiable Graphics created beautiful playbills. My comedian friend Erin Rosaire helped direct. To this day, I feel so blessed that these individuals helped me put this show together. It was very rewarding, I must say. Charitable organizations need more people to organize such events. Challenge yourself in a charitable way.

EXERCISES

(1) Which charity or charities do I wish to donate to?

(2) What type of event can I put together for this charity to attract donations and participation?

TOOL 107. DO A RANDOM ACT OF KINDNESS

Not everything in life has a price tag on it. We get to experience things in life that are priceless. A random act of kindness is doing something for someone else just because you feel like bringing sunshine to their day. Your act of kindness is done without expectations for anything in return.

In modern-day society, engaging in a random act of kindness is not common. Why? My theory is simple: people are too preoccupied with the things in life that aren't important. We are always rushing to go from here to there and everywhere. This fast-paced society has created many hypnotized and over-involved minds. We lack *presence* when it really matters. Can you imagine being *present* and not being so much in a rush all the time? For example, you may discover someone fighting tears behind you in line at a coffee shop. You can whisper to the cashier, "And I've got them covered for a four-dollar coffee or whatever they want." A random act of kindness for a person in need can turn around someone's entire day. You can literally wipe their tears away.

Being conscious of your surroundings is the solution to slowing down the fast pace we've adopted as Americans. It's up to us to relearn what it truly means to be an attentive person. Our bodies are not designed to be moving at a constantly fast pace. Losing weight requires a more moderate pace. This is why I mentioned in tool 26 that you should learn how to march to your own beat.

Random acts of kindness help you build a higher level of self-love. When you love yourself, you're able to love others and be the stable force in their lives. The love that people feel for you should be the love that you feel for yourself.

Go above and beyond by offering other human beings something they would never expect. Be their angel for the day. Random acts don't always have to cost you money. Below are some ideas for random acts of kindness:

- Tell someone you like their outfit today.

- Tell someone you love their smile.

- Open the door for someone.

- Hold the elevator for someone.

- Smile at someone.

- Buy someone a glass of wine at a restaurant.

- Buy someone their coffee.

- Buy breakfast for a homeless person.

- Give the cable guy a bottled water to take on the road.

- Tip your server extra cash for any service that went above and beyond your expectations.

- Place a chocolate heart on all the desks at work to show your appreciation for your colleagues.

- Write someone a thank-you card.

- Write someone a positive e-mail.

- Call someone back in a timely fashion despite your schedule demands.

- Share your expertise with someone at no cost.

One act of kindness I've mastered is that I always write letters of commendation for people in the service industry who go above and beyond my expectations. One day at Staples, the cashier set me up on one of their laptops across the store to print out my coupons, since I didn't have mine with me. I was able to save ten dollars as a result of her act of kindness. Who gives this type of service these days? I made it very clear to her that she'd made my day. She loved hearing that. Since I have an extensive background in management, I know it's valuable to provide an employee with positive feedback for their human resources file, too. Many employees do not make a lot of money, so why not reward them with appreciative words regarding your personal experience with them? If it was a great experience, let someone know. This may get them a raise or even save their job. Take an extra three minutes out of your day to tell their manager how great your experience was in front of the employee. People love to feel validated and deserve to be validated when they exceed your expectations.

Let your weight-loss success be your own random act of kindness to yourself every day by committing to patience, perseverance, and love for yourself until you hit your goal. No more giving up, quitting, or being impatient with the process. It's completely in your power to succeed—I believe in you!

EXERCISES

(1) What is one random act of kindness that I did today?

(2) How did the person respond?

(3) What random act did I do for myself today?

(4) How did it make me feel?

CONCLUSION

I remember one day, when I was writing this book, I stopped for a moment, turned to G-d, and said, "Oh my G-d, I'm writing a book—an amazing book!" I hope you feel you've read an amazing book. Please use the tools presented in this book to help you unlock your potential in becoming a healthier person. I understand your frustrations with weight loss. Please realize you may not find that all the tools work for you all of the time. That's okay. Find a tool in this book every time you open it, and start mastering that tool each day. I hope you will turn to the tools as often as you need them throughout your journey.

Realize that you have a choice of the type of life you live. The more in tuned you are with your journey, the more powerful your journey will become. This will ultimately lead you to a place of self-realization; a feeling of being triumphant. Along the way, you'll meet lots of great people, realize how great you are, and maximize your full potential. Don't let anyone in your life bring you down. You deserve the most rewarding life of all, and that is a life full of love and good health. Spread the joy of being healthy to those you love. Believe in yourself and realize that it's up to you to break your chains of being overweight. Your individual journey is part of the bigger picture in helping me break the chains of obesity in America.

To a healthy, lean, and invigorated you!

XO, JZ

Smile and Believe
www.JZfitness.com
jz@jzfitness.com

SUGGESTED READING

Consider reading some additional literature on many of the topics discussed in my book.

1) Apovian, C. "Sugar-sweetened Soft Drinks, Obesity, and Type 2 Diabetes." *JAMA* 292(8): 978–979.

2) Arhant-Sudhir K., R. Arhant-Sudhir, and K. Sudhir. "Pet Ownership and Cardiovascular Risk Reduction: Supporting Evidence, Conflicting Data and Underlying Mechanisms." *Clinical and Experimental Pharmacology and Physiology* 38(11) (2011): 734–8.

3) Avena, N. M. "Evidence for Sugar Addiction: Behavioral and Neurochemical Effects of Intermittent, Excessive Sugar Intake." *Neuroscience & Biobehavioral Reviews,* 32(1) (2008): 20–39.

4) Barnes, D., and C. Yaffe. "The Projected Effect of Risk Factor Reduction on Alzheimer's Disease Prevalence." *The Lancet Neurology* 10(9) (2011): 819–828.

5) Benedict, H. "A Biometric Study of Human Basal Metabolism." *PNAS USA* 4(12): 370–373.

6) Bleich, S., Y. Wang, Y. Wang, and S. Gortmaker. "Increasing Consumption of Sugar-sweetened Beverages among U.S. Adults." *American Journal of Clinical Nutrition.* 89(1) (2009): 372-381.

7) Block, Stanley H., "You Don't Have to Get Rid of Cravings." *Come to Your Senses* (blog), *Psychology*

Today, July 27, 2011, http://www.psychology-today.com/blog/come-your-senses/201107/you-dont-have-get-rid-cravings.

8) Brown, D. and Gordon, G. Detox with Oral Chelation: Protecting Yourself from Lead, Mercury and Other Environmental Toxins. Smart Publications, 2009.

9) Ceriello, A. "Oxidative Stress and Glycemic Regulation." *Metabolism* 49(2 Suppl1) (Feb 2000): 27–29.

10) Christakis, Nicholas A., and James H. Fowler. "The Spread of Obesity in a Large Social Network over 32 Years." *New England Journal of Medicine* 357: 370–379, http://content.nejm.org/cgi/content/full/357/4/370?query=TOC.

11) Davis, J. "Detox Diets: Cleansing the Body—Spring Cleaning, A WebMD Feature," http://www.webmd.com/diet/features/detox-diets-cleansing-body.

12) Edlund, Matthew. "Diet and Exercise Won't Solve Obesity." *The Power of Rest* (blog), *Psychology Today,* June 2, 2011, http://www.psychologytoday.com/blog/the-power-rest/201106/diet-and-exercise-wont-solve-obesity.

13) Edwards, Betty. *Drawing on the Right Side of the Brain.* Penguin Putnam Inc., 1980.

14) "Food Label Helps Consumers Make Healthier Choices," FDA, http://www.fda.gov/ForConsumers/ConsumerUpdates/ucm094536.html.

15) Furth, A. and J. Harding. "Why Sugar Is Bad For You." *New Scientist* (September 23, 1989): 44.

16) Garrison, R., and E. Somer. *The Nutrition Desk Reference.* New Canaan: Keats Publishing, 1985.

17) Glinsmann, W., et al. "Evaluation of Health Aspects of Sugar Contained in Carbohydrate Sweeteners." FDA Report of Sugars Task Force (1986): 39.

18) Grontved, A., and F. Hu. "Television Viewing and Risk of Type 2 Diabetes, Cardiovascular Disease, and All-Cause Mortality: A Meta-analysis." *JAMA* 305(23): 2448–2455.

19) Hertoghe, T. *The Hormone Handbook*, 2nd ed. Luxemburg: International Medical Books, 2010: 43–52.

20) Katz, Terese Weinstein. "Should You Call Yourself a Food Addict?" *Thin from Within* (blog), *Psychology Today,* April 19, 2011, http://www.psychologytoday.com/blog/thin-within/201104/should-you-call-yourself-food-addict.

21) Laursen P., and Jenkins, D. "The Scientific Basis for High-intensity Interval Training: Optimizing Training Programs and Maximizing Performance in Highly Trained Endurance Athletes." *Sports Medicine* 32(1): 53–73.

22) Lee, A. T., and Cerami, A. "The Role of Glycation in Aging." *Annals of the New York Academy of Sciences,* (1992) 663: 63–70.

23) Lohman, E. B., J. S. Petrofsky, C. Maloney-Hinds, H. Betts-Schwab, and D. Thorpe. "The Effect of Whole Body Vibration on Lower Extremity Skin Blood Flow in Normal Subjects." *Medical Science Monitor* 13(2): CR71–76.

24) Ludwig, D. S., et al. "High Glycemic Index Foods, Overeating, and Obesity." *Pediatrics*, 103(3) (March 1999): 26-32.

25) Medline Plus. "Fish Oil: Natural Medicines Comprehensive Database Consumer Version." http://www.nlm.nih.gov/medlineplus/druginfo/natural/993.html.

26) Meyer, P., et al. Interval training: Can it boost your calorie-burning power? 2009, http://www.mayoclinic.com/health/interval-training/SM00110

27) Mifflin, St. J., et al. "A New Predictive Equation for Resting Energy Expenditure in Healthy Individuals." *American Journal of Clinical Nutrition (1990)* 51(2): 241–247.

28) Montana State University, Bozeman. "Performance Benchmarks—Body Composition and Body Mass." http://btc.montana.edu/olympics/physiology/pb03.html.

29) Office of the Surgeon General. "The Surgeon General's Call to Action to Prevent and Decrease Overweight and Obesity," 2007, http://www.surgeongeneral.gov/topics/obesity/calltoaction/fact_adolescents.htm.

30) O'Sullivan, J., and C. Mahan. "Blood Sugar Levels, Glycosuria, and Body Weight Related to Development of Diabetes Mellitus: The Oxford Epidemiologic Study 17 Years Later." *JAMA* 194(6): 587–592.

31) Pereira, M. "Obesity Epidemiology." *JAMA*, 301(21): 2274–2275.

32) Pierpaoli, W., and W. Regelson. *The Melatonin Miracle.* New York: Simon & Schuster, 1995.

33) Pretlow, Robert, MD. *Overweight: What Kids Say: What's Really Causing the Childhood Obesity Epidemic.* CreateSpace, 2010.

34) The Regence Group. "Medical Policy," accessed on August 10, 2011, http://blue.regence.com/trgmedpol/radiology/rad41.html.

35) Schmitz K., P. J. Hannan, S. D. Stovitz, C. J. Bryan, M. Warren, et al. "Strength Training and Adiposity in Premenopausal Women: Strong, Healthy, and Empowered Study." *American Journal of Clinical Nutrition* 86: 566–572.

36) Science Daily. "Coffee, Energy Drinkers Beware: Many Mega-Sized Drinks Loaded with Sugar, Nutrition Expert Says," February 3, 2011, http://www.sciencedaily.com/releases/2011/02/110203124820.htm.

37) Shape Up America! "Shape Up and Drop 10."

38) http://www.shapeup.org/atmstd/sud10v3/sud10s7.php.

39) Sizer, F., and E. Whitney. *Nutrition Concepts and Controversies,* 9th ed. (Belmont: Wadsworth, 2003): 105.

40) http://www.sleepfoundation.org

41) *"SMART Criteria"*: *http*://en.wikipedia.org/wiki/SMART_criteria

42) Tsai, A., and T. Wadden. "Systematic Review: An Evaluation of Major Commercial Weight Loss

Programs in the United States." *Annals of Internal Medicine* 142: 56–66.

43) Vastag, B. "Obesity Is Now on Everyone's Plate." *JAMA* 291(10): 1186–88.

44) Welch, J. *Winning*. New York: Harper Collins Business Publishers, 2005.

45) Vissers, D., A. Verrijken, I. Mertens, C. van Gils, A. van de Sompel, S. Truijen, and L. Van Gaal. Effect of Long-term Whole Body Vibration Training on Visceral Adipose Tissue: A Preliminary Report. Obesity facts." Pub Med, 2007, http://www.ncbi.nlm.nih.gov/pubmed/20484941.

NOTES

Made in the USA
San Bernardino, CA
12 December 2014